CHRONIC
PAIN
CHRONICLES

INSIGHTFUL AND INSPIRING STORIES OF
RESOLVE, RESILIENCE, AND RELIEF

MDG BOOKS

Philadelphia, Pennsylvania

©2025 MEDIA DEVELOPMENT GROUP LLC. ALL RIGHTS RESERVED.
ISBN: 979-8-218-82511-9

Contents

I wrote this book after years of experiencing, researching, and pondering chronic pain

We are bonded by the barriers we've faced

Genetic testing uncovered the cause of my chronic pain — and troubling questions

A pain sufferer and "metagerontologist" helps others navigate our maddening healthcare system

Dashed dreams, lost purpose, and damaged finances go with job loss due to pain

The bill for pain to US society and sufferers is more than $722 billion a year

Those of us with chronic pain struggle with constant stress

A newly graduated graphic artist hates to think about living the rest of her life in pain

Praise for *Chronic Pain Chronicles*

Courageous. Insightful. Heartbreaking. Hopeful. From the perspective of his own unimaginable pain, and in interviews with others in constant pain, Randall H. Duckett delivers an expertly written, highly readable science-backed handbook for chronic pain sufferers that is both instructional and motivational, packed with under-appreciated challenges and lesser-known remedies. Anyone with ongoing pain will glean inspiration to carry on and strategies to alleviate their suffering.

—*Robert Roy Britt, founder and editor of* Wise & Well *and author of* Make Sleep Your Superpower

Chronic Pain Chronicles *completely transformed my perspective on pain. Randall H. Duckett has succeeded in packing a life's worth of insights into this book. It helped me understand what's happening with some of my closest friends who are suffering from chronic pain — behaviors I had little insight into before reading it. I learned to have more compassion for everything they're dealing with — physically, mentally, socially, and spiritually. I'm taking the lessons I've learned to hopefully become a better friend.*

— *Kathleen Murphy, independent health journalist*

Dedication

Chronic Pain Chronicles is dedicated to Jamie, Lane, Sean, Jen, Josh, Ryan, Chris, Liz, and all the other physical therapists who worked so hard to help me rehab and get stronger.

To the doctors, physician assistants, nurses, and other healthcare providers who gave me expert care.

And to my family — particularly my pushy wife, MeK — who help me live a wonderful life despite my disabilities.

Notes

Thank you for reading *Chronic Pain Chronicles: Insightful and inspiring stories of resolve, resilience, and relief.* Here are a few notes to keep in mind:

> *"I am not a physician or other healthcare professional."*

- Important: I am not a physician or any other healthcare professional. I am a chronic pain sufferer and a journalist covering the topic of chronic pain. You should always consult a qualified physician or other medical professional before starting, continuing, or ceasing any treatment.

- This is not a medical book. It is a work of reporting and commentary intended to educate, entertain, and enlighten readers about what it's like to live in chronic pain. If you follow the advice from me, those people quoted, or from other sources, always make sure it is right for you by consulting an experienced, licensed healthcare professional beforehand.

- Warning: The book's content may touch on difficult subjects, including suicide. If something in this book negatively affects you, please stop reading immediately and get help. 24/7 assistance can be reached by calling or texting 988 at the 988 Suicide & Crisis Lifeline. You can also text 741741.

- To the best of my knowledge, information is correct at the time of writing. For links to sources, see the e-book edition. You are urged to ensure they are current before you quote, use, or otherwise cite them in any format. I regret any errors, typos, or other mistakes in this book. Corrections can be found at randallhduckett.com.

- Direct quotes are indicated either by quotation marks or indentation and italics. Quotes and other information have been copyedited to match the *Chronic Pain Chronicles* style guide and for spelling, grammar, clarity, and brevity. Quotes are the opinions of the sources and not necessarily the perspectives of the author, staff, or publisher.

- Versions of the chapters, profiles, and other information in this book first appeared on Medium.com, username @rhduckett234. I invite you to read my further reporting on chronic pain, aging, and other topics there.

- I hope you find this book valuable and enjoyable. If so, please rate and review it on Amazon, Good Reads, and other book sites. Five-star ratings and thoughtful reviews are much appreciated.

- Please visit randallhduckett.com to ask questions, make comments, or contact me. I'd love to comment about chronic pain for media outlets such as YouTube videos or podcasts.

- I hope you enjoy *Chronic Pain Chronicles* and gain valuable information, insight, and inspiration from it.

Foreword

Pain's Mind-Body Connection

By Dr. Andrea Furlan

In 1995, the *British Medical Journal (BMJ)* reported the case of a 29-year-old construction worker who was rushed to the emergency department after falling onto a 6-inch nail. It went all the way through his boot and the tip was visible on the top.

He was stunned and terrified. Any small movement caused terrible pain, so doctors had to give him fentanyl (a powerful painkiller) and midazolam to sedate him before they pulled the nail out from the sole.

When the boot was removed, doctors noticed there was no blood and the worker's skin was intact. The nail had passed harmlessly between his toes. No physical damage had been done, yet he still felt excruciating pain.

> *"If the pain system can be activated just by believing there is a threat, it can also be deactivated."*

Who's to say that his pain was not real? It was, but the worker did not need painful physical damage to feel it — there was none. All he needed was the pain centers in his brain to become activated.

This is actually good news, because it shows that if the pain system can be activated just by believing there is a threat, it can also be deactivated by believing that the threat is removed.

This real-life story illustrates something that many people do not know about pain: that pain isn't just about physical damage. It is also about expectations formed by one's conscious and unconscious mind, a person's memory, attitudes, values, and experiences.

"Pain affects about one in five individuals worldwide."

As a pain specialist for the more than 30 years, I have seen firsthand how chronic pain can be devastating to individuals, to their families, friends, and to society. I am a MD, PhD, professor of medicine at the University of Toronto, and author of *8 Steps to Conquer Chronic Pain: A Doctor's Guide to Lifelong Relief.* I've created scores of videos explaining chronic pain on my YouTube channel (@DrAndreaFurlan) and on my website (doctorandreafurlan.com).

Pain affects about one in five individuals worldwide, including children. I have helped many people to overcome and conquer their pain by thinking about it differently and making lifestyle changes, but it is up to each of my patients to put my advice into practice.

What I ask of them is very simple, but they might be the most challenging steps for them: retrain their brain, control their emotions, get quality sleep, adjust their diet, seek help from others, reduce their medication use, exercise more, and focus on their goals.

Pain is a biopsychosocial construct shaped in the brain. The brain's function is to preserve the status quo, and it does this by predicting the future (the next second, minute, day, year, etc.). Like in the case of the construction worker, when the brain perceives "danger" (whether real or not), it triggers an alarm, which can manifest as pain. Sometimes it may also trigger extreme fatigue, dizziness, tremors, a heart palpitation, or shortness of breath. We cannot separate the body from the mind, or pain from our emotions. It is impossible to conquer pain, especially chronic pain, if the person suffering pain does not recognize these relationships. The first step to conquer chronic pain is to understand it.

Reading *Chronic Pain Chronicles* by Randall H. Duckett brought back memories of hundreds of stories I've heard from my patients over the past more than three decades of practicing as a pain doctor. Randall is both an accomplished journalist and lifelong pain sufferer, and this unique combination makes his book both a pleasure to read and a fascinating learning journey. Writing about one's own suffering and emotional battles is never easy, yet Randall does so with openness, poetry, self-awareness, and compassion. This work is more than just a valuable resource for people living with chronic pain, or the autobiography of someone enduring persistent and frustrating discomfort. It is also a profound chronicling of the experience of having chronic pain. For that, I warmly congratulate Randall. I think you'll find his book as enlightening as I did. Enjoy.

Part I: Chronicling My Chronic Pain

"Turn your wounds into wisdom."

— Oprah Winfrey

"No one saves us but ourselves. No one can and no one may. We ourselves must walk the path."

—Buddha

"These pains you feel are messengers. Listen to them."

— Rumi

Source: Wisdomquotes.com

1

Painful Words

I wrote this book after years of experiencing, researching, and pondering chronic pain

They say, "Write about what you know."

I know pain.

When it comes to hurt, I have a PhD (Personal history of Disease).

This is a book about my life in pain, but it's much more. It also features stories from other sufferers (see Pain Profiles and Pain Points). It offers reporting about chronic pain, including advice from experts and the latest research into it. It's designed to capture what it's like to live in chronic pain and, if you are a fellow sufferer, to help you feel understood and less alone.

MY STORY

Diagnosed at age 6, I suffer from a rare genetic condition called multiple epiphyseal dysplasia (MED), which caused my joints and bones to deform as I grew and aged.

I share this rare distinction — MED occurs in about one out of every 20,000 births — with *It's Always Sunny in Philadelphia* actor and Jersey Mike's pitchman Danny DeVito (though I am of average height as compared to his 4'11" frame) and former Secretary of Labor Robert Reich.

To understand MED's effect on my body, think of broken gears constantly grinding against each

*"[Pain is] an unpleasant sensory and emotional experience associated with, or resembling that associated with, actual or potential tissue damage."
—International Association for the Study of Pain (IASP)*

other and wearing down with use. Over time, this has resulted in osteoarthritis and severe chronic pain (technically known as chronic pain syndrome).

Every day, I ache head to toe, mostly with osteoarthritis in my legs, torso, arms, and neck. I get frequent stress headaches and jaw pain, likely from the tension of girding myself against hurt. I suffer from comorbidities that go with pain, like depression (see chapter 10) and anxiety. I have neuropathy in my lower legs and scoliosis, stenosis, and bone spurs in my lower back. My left foot constantly spasms due to nerve damage from an ankle fusion. My right elbow freezes up frequently and I sometimes have a pain in my left hip from some leftover hardware from a hip replacement. My tail bone gets painful when I sit on hard surfaces, which was caused by years of slouching in a wheelchair.

Pain infuses my body, which feels like a sponge dipped in acid.

EXAMINING MY PAIN

Ack! Enough complaining. I'm not a whiner. I tell you all this not to get sympathy, but to establish my bona fides as someone who knows what it's like to have chronic pain. Throughout the years, I've done an untold number of things to control my pain and find relief.

I've had eight joint replacements (both hips twice, both knees, and both shoulders) plus had both my ankles fused. I have more metal in me than the X-Man Wolverine (played in the movies by Hugh Jackman), whose skeleton is laced with the indestructible and fictional metal adamantium. (See comic books and movies.)

I've taken thousands of pills and used countless opioids (see chapter 7). I've done dozens of procedures like injections and epidurals. I spent hundreds of hours doing physical therapy. I've tried everything from complicated knee braces to a TENS unit, which sends electronic pluses to disrupt pain signals.

I've lived with chronic pain for decades, but until a couple of years ago, I didn't really examine it. For all my experience with hurt, l didn't know a lot about it.

It was just a given, a part of my life. It had brought extreme consequences, including crashing my career (see chapter 4) and forcing me to retire at age 53 due to disability. It cost me an estimated $2 million (see chapter 5). It affected my relationships with my wife (see chapter 2). As I aged, it threatened to take over my life.

In late 2023, after a decade of surgeries (see chapter 4), I felt well enough to apply my skills as a journalist of 40 years experience to studying chronic pain — mine and that of others. The result of my research and thinking is this book.

A WHOLE LOT OF HURT GOING ON

It took me about two seconds of googling to discover I am not alone in my pain.

According to the National Center for Health Statistics, "In 2023, 24.3% of adults had chronic pain, and 8.5% of adults had chronic pain that … limited life or work activities (referred to as high impact chronic pain or HICP) in the past 3 months." Doing the math, that translates to more than 60 million American adults with chronic pain. That's about twice the population of Texas. About 21 million have HICP — more than the number of folks who live in Florida.

What's most astounding is how pain has skyrocketed recently. A previous report from the Centers for Disease Control and Prevention (CDC) showed that the rate of chronic pain stayed relatively steady between 2016 (20.4%) and 2021 (20.9%), then shot up by 3% in just two years (2021 to 2023). That's 8,670,000 more American adults who reported chronic pain. This time correlates to the pandemic, of course. Whether the rate of increase will continue is unknown.

And it's not just adults in enduring hurt. According to the journal *Pain*, in the 70 countries studied: "The overall prevalence of chronic pain in children and adolescents was 20.8%, with the highest prevalence for headache and musculoskeletal pain (25.7%)."

"Acute pain happens suddenly, starts out sharp or intense, and serves as a warning sign of disease or threat to the body. It is caused by injury, surgery, illness, trauma, or painful medical procedures and generally lasts from a few minutes to less than six months. Acute pain usually disappears whenever the underlying cause is treated or healed."
— IASP

That means one in five kids is in chronic pain. As a lifelong sufferer, I can testify that pain in childhood shapes you as a person.

Digging into the numbers, chronic pain is more prevalent in females (see chapter 19), in older people, and in rural communities.

> *"Chronic pain is pain that persists or recurs for longer than three months."*
> *— IASP*

The CDC also reports:

- Pain is the number-one reason Americans use the healthcare system.

- Chronic pain is the leading cause of long-term disability in the United States.

- Chronic pain disproportionally affects the poor.

Chronic pain has an impact on us all, not just its sufferers. A 2010 estimate found that America spends up to a whopping $635 billion each year on chronic pain in terms of medical treatments, disability payments, and lost productivity. That's a 15-year-old number, so I'd wager that the economic impact of chronic pain in 2025 is about $1 trillion annually (see chapter 5).

The legions of people with chronic pain and their loved ones and healthcare professionals who tend to them is predicted by the National Institutes of Health (NIH) to grow in coming years due in part to an aging American population, the prevalence of long COVID-19, and better understanding of how chronic pain really works. (NIH referred to it as its own separate disease in 2005).

NUMBERS DON'T TELL THE STORY

Some 60 million people (including 21 million of them with HICP) represent enormous numbers, yet they, by themselves, don't tell the story of chronic pain.

That's because these stats represent tens of millions of individual people who hurt. This may be you, your family members, your friends, your coworkers, or others you know. The gross numbers belie the suffering that these folks endure — the aches, stabs, zaps, burning, soreness, stinging, pangs, agony, anguish, searing, misery, torture, and more that make up the lexicon of symptoms of chronic pain.

Exaggeration? The impact is not only physical, but mental. Think about what it must be to feel trapped in your own body, at the mercy of pain that's often out of control, hurt that doesn't heal, hurt that's permanent.

Some conditions might be merely irritating, like a hitch in the hip, but can drive a person crazy, like having flies constantly buzz in your ear.

Some are excruciating, like extreme lower back pain (the most common kind of chronic pain), and leaves sufferers confined to their chair or bed.

There is not one kind of chronic pain because there is not one kind of human. Each person's pain is unique. I cannot feel your pain and you cannot feel mine.

Those of us who suffer from chronic pain are caged in our bodies with a hungry tiger stalking us. Not only is there physical danger; there is mental anguish as we, being human, try to think of solutions to our pain, ways that will make it more survivable, ways to outfox and "fix" it.

THE BRAIN IS FLEXIBLE

But pain is a cruel opponent.

The nature of chronic pain, though, is that it often can't be completely cured. It may be eased by medication, operations, and other treatments, but, by definition, it endures. Most often, it cannot be fixed in the conventional sense of completely going away. It can only be managed.

That is not to say there is no hope. Emerging science sees chronic pain as an aberration of the body, biology gone wrong, but more so, it's something that happens in the brain, where pain is perceived (see chapter 15).

More research has uncovered that the brain is flexible, which is called "neuroplasticity." As such, conscious thoughts and conditioned responses can be manipulated.

In short, the brain is where pain is processed. It can decide pain is agonizing or it can take it away. In fact, some have retrained their brains to cure chronic pain (see Pain Profile: Cured By Brain Retraining).

The advice to sufferers I hear most often, from patients to experts, is to not give up. Chronic pain can be conquered.

THOUGHTS ON PAIN

Why did I call this book *Chronic Pain Chronicles*? It speaks to the diverse feelings sufferers have about being hurt, the many stories that go with pain. The aim of the book is to answer a simple question: What does living in chronic pain really feel like?

In the following pages, you'll find essays on various aspects of chronic pain, from its mechanism (see chapter 15) to how to reach acceptance (see chapter 36). These essays reflect my unique perspective on pain. But I've found they are topics others can relate to, common feelings that span sufferers.

"I cannot feel your pain and you cannot feel mine."

At its essence: *Chronic Pain Chronicles* offers perspectives on pain from me and many other sources. Its core is my life story and those of people who suffer, along with thoughts from doctors, physical therapists, and other experts who work with such people. I hope they offer information, insight, and inspiration.

ESSAY SOURCE

Versions of these essays first were published on Medium.com, an online site where writers and readers come together to share news, perspective, and thinking. I spent all of 2024 and the first half of 2025 researching and reporting on chronic pain — mine and that of others. These essays have been edited and slightly rewritten for this book. (For my latest work, follow me on Medium @randall234.)

Medium welcomes users to comment on pieces like mine, so many of the ones here include what I call Pain Points, thoughts from other sufferers that add to what I've written. Commentators are identified by their Medium usernames unless otherwise requested.

Throughout this book, I've also done Pain Profiles of people in chronic pain, from a graphic designer in her 20s (see Pain Profile: Craving Relief) to an amateur poet in her 60s (see Pain Profile: Game Pain). I'm grateful to these folks for sharing their stories.

I AM NOT A DOCTOR

It is important to note that this is not a medical book (and I am not a doctor or healthcare provider).

This is also not a science book. I urge you to learn more about the technical aspects of pain from the sources I've included, but you do not need to know them to understand this book.

I interviewed experts, but there are plenty of books about pain by people with letters after their names.

Precious few are from actual sufferers, and those tend to be memoirs rather than reporting on pain. With this book, I've tried to give sufferers a voice.

As you read further, you'll get different slices of the chronic pain story.

- If you are a sufferer, *Chronic Pain Chronicles* is aimed at helping better understand pain by exploring key aspects of what it's like and offering advice about how to cope. It will give hope to sufferers and help them feel less alone (loneliness is a common complaint; see chapter 16).

- If you are a caregiver or loved one of a chronic pain sufferer, you'll find a window on the chronic pain and come to better understand what people for whom you care are going through.

- If you are a physician, nurse, or other healthcare provider, you'll come to better grasp where patients are coming from, where the healthcare system fails them, what can be improved.

- If you are a policymaker, you'll see that there are real people out there suffering and deserving assistance, not by restrictions on medications but proactive programs to help constituents trapped in their bodies, feeling forgotten.

The book is unique in the chronic pain self-help genre, in that it is about the fierce feelings that come with chronic pain, including the powerful mind-body connection (see Foreword). Physical pain affects emotions and vice versa.

After a long debate with myself about just what to call us, I use the word "sufferer" in this book to describe people in chronic pain.

"Patient" is too clinical and impersonal. The term doesn't capture anything near the experience of pain, other than that lots of us spend too many hours in waiting rooms being impatient patients.

We should not be defined by our pathologies. I hate it when doctors and nurses say things like, "Oh, you're the hip" rather than referring to me as a person.

I haven't found a better word than *sufferer*. To me, it gets closest to the experience of people in chronic pain — we are indeed suffering.

WHY ME?
Why should you listen to me?

In short: My expertise is my experience.

Not only have I lived a lifetime of pain, I am a journalist who's expert at research and storytelling. Just because I was forced to retire relatively young (see chapter 4) doesn't mean I lost my journalism skills.

"My expertise is my experience."

I've also done years of research for this book. I've read hundreds of stories about chronic pain from dozens of publications. I have more than 125,000 words of research in one Word file and I've collected published stories of people in pain in another. I've spent hours in online chronic pain groups like those on Facebook and Reddit. I've attended scores of Zoom support groups, most often those offered by the U.S. Pain Foundation (see Sources of Solace). I've written columns for the America Chronic Pain Association's quarterly e-magazine. I've interviewed dozens of sufferers and experts who have generously shared their perspectives on pain. This book is like a dissertation, my report on chronic pain.

If you find *Chronic Pain Chronicles* valuable, tell others. Do an online review and rate it five stars. Gift it to those you know in pain and to their caretakers. Send it to your government representatives. Let's get the word out that chronic pain is a gigantic problem and tens of millions of us need help dealing with it.

Also, please visit my website at randallhduckett.com to see comments on *Chronic Pain Chronicles* and learn more about chronic pain.

My motivation to do this book is simple: I wanted to understand my pain better. But there was another reason. I, like many chronic pain sufferers, feel very alone in my pain. It's hard to imagine that there are others feeling the same things I feel, having similar experiences, living like lives. But, indeed, there are tens of millions who are. I researched, wrote, edited, and published this book to help me feel less alone, which it has.

I hope you feel less alone, too.

2

My Pushy Wife

We are bonded by the barriers we've faced

This was it: I would die at the hands of a taxi in Istanbul.

My wife, whose nickname is MeK (me-kay), inched me out as we strove to cross a car-clogged street in the city where Europe ends and Asia begins.

This apparently offended the drivers of yellow cabs who refused to cede to us. Sitting in my wheelchair — which had made the 5,644 mile trip (as the crow flies) with us from our then home in Knoxville, Tennessee, to Turkey's largest city — I felt out of control as the notorious traffic bore down. At the last nanosecond, MeK snatched my chair backward, saving me.

> *"MeK's willingness to push me has opened up more new adventures than my health should allow."*

The ancient world — Istanbul was founded as Constantinople 1,800 years ago — wasn't built for people with disabilities. In the city of 15.4 million, my wife maneuvered me as she struggled down ripped-up sidewalks and brutally bumpy cobblestone streets. She carried the wheelchair up the railless stairs to the second-story apartment where we stayed. She hefted it into the trunks of taxis whose drivers were clearly suspicious of a handicapped American.

Still, together with my wheelchair, my able-bodied wife and I rolled through the Hagia Sophia (which dates from the 6th century), back when it was a secular museum and not the working mosque it now is. Thanks to helpful young Turks and a lift, we were able to weave through the Basilica Cistern, an underground reservoir with its 336 columns, two supported by partially submerged Medusa heads. We braved the Spice Bazaar, where disaster nearly struck again. At one point, we encountered a downhill grade. My wife used every bit of her 115 pounds to hold back her 200-plus-pound husband from mowing down a group of women in burkas.

Over the years before and since then, MeK's willingness to push me has opened up more new adventures than my health should allow. She has become expert at sussing out accessible places — state and national parks with paved trails, nature preserves with boardwalks, beaches with concrete pathways to the sand.

She looks out for me, always scanning ahead to what's coming. She has become an expert at turning the wheelchair backward to get over large humps and cracks in streets and sidewalks. Seeking accessibility, we often discover new places even locals don't know.

> *"My wife of nearly 40 years … has been there through all the ups and downs of the hospital stays, rehabs, and opioids."*

CARING CAREGIVER

When I was just 53, I was forced to retire from my career in journalism and marketing (see chapter 4) when both my feet became frozen at 45-degree angles to the ankles, causing me to walk, when I could, on the outside edges. Another pair of fusions corrected this condition.

In the 2010s, I had seven operations in seven years, the last a gastric sleeve to curb my ballooning obesity, which was hard on my failing joints. Another reason: My petite wife increasingly had trouble with handling my hefty weight in the wheelchair, particularly when we went uphill.

All the while, my wife propelled me — figuratively and literally — to recover. She wheeled me to physical therapy appointments and physician's offices. She emptied the urinal when I was laid up from the joint replacements. She weighed my food and gave me protein shakes after the bariatric surgery, as I lost a more wheelchair-manageable 80 pounds.

My wife of nearly 40 years, if we make it to 2026, has been there through all the ups and downs of the hospital stays, rehabs, and opioids. When I couldn't walk, she didn't walk.

HAVING MY BACK

Now in my 60s, I walk with a cane around the house and for short distances, often using MeK's shoulder to steady my gait. We break the wheelchair out of the back of our SUV when we get out and about.

To cope with my disability, I spend my life trying to stay in control. Each step and movement are fraught because of the pain they can cause. I spend my days anticipating physical and emotional danger (see chapter 6). I like to think that if I can just control my environment, I can fend off the worst parts of being disabled.

But in the wheelchair, I have no control. When we travel, I depend on MeK to have my back, literally. Like that day in Istanbul, I've had to give up control and trust her implicitly to get me safely where I need to go.

I fret that I'm imposing on her too much, that I am somehow forcing her — the old "in-sickness-and-in-health" vow we made back in the '80s — to give up a part of herself to care for me. Would she, I often wonder, be better off not pushing me around? I usually repress such feelings, but I asked MeK about them.

"I love pushing you," she responded from the kitchen as I sat in my La-Z-Boy in the living room of our home in suburban Philadelphia. "Pushing you feels like we're walking together. It's made me more conscious of my surroundings. I have such great memories of exploring with you."

The only thing she dislikes about pushing, MeK adds, is that unless she puts her Apple Watch in her pocket to capture the motion of moving, rather on her wrist resting on the wheelchair handles, she fails to get credit toward the 10,000 steps she shoots for everyday.

Sure, sometimes MeK pushes my buttons. I get defensive when I perceive she's judging me. That comes from a lifetime of being embarrassed by being different and trying in vain to control my image as a "perfect" person.

I get ashamed of being in the chair and unable to walk on my own two feet. I hate it when strangers on the street judge me as being an invalid. I cringe when I have to ask them to step aside to let my wheelchair through.

MeK never makes me feel bad about being disabled, however. I know that minding a handicapped person is hard on her body and emotions. When I get upset, I try to remember that pushing the wheelchair and other acts of care-giving is her love language. She does it for the life we've built over four decades of knowing each other and being best friends.

We are bonded by the barriers we've faced.

One of my favorite quotes, from U2's Bono about his long marriage with his wife, Ali, sums up our symbiotic relationship: "A shared life gives you a shared memory. She's my witness. I'm hers."

Pain Points

"I've a history with a bad knee and leg problems — and with travel! Fortunately, I only needed wheelchair assistance in airports (where my wife benefited by joining me at the head of the security and Customs lines), but otherwise, she was my legs in scouting around and in other ways. Now I get along pretty well but use a walking stick for longer jaunts (like airports). Sometimes I miss the wheelchair express, but not enough to go back to that. The stick does grant similar privileges. On our last couple of trips we were in long airport lines and my wife said, 'Stick your stick out there where they can see it.' Sure enough, we were ushered to the shortest lines. I am not proud — or ashamed!"
—J. Avery Stewart

Pain Points are comments on this essay as it appeared originally on Medium.com. They are solely the opinions of the commentators and do not necessarily reflect the views of the book author or publisher.

3

DNA Dilemma

*Genetic testing uncovered the cause of my chronic pain —
and troubling questions*

I am a mutant.

And not the cool kind who can shoot lasers from his eyes or phase through walls.

No, my mutation doesn't make me a superhero. In fact, it's a villain to me. My mutated genes have caused me severe chronic pain from head to toe. As I grew from childhood, my joints and bones deformed, leading to osteoarthritis throughout the body. This led to multiple joint replacement operations on my knees, hips, and shoulders. I also had my ankles fused.

I have a rare disease called multiple epiphyseal dysplasia (MED). In my early childhood in Los Angeles, my mother recognized I couldn't walk correctly, so she took me to a Beverly Hills orthopedist. The team doctor for what was that era's Oakland Raiders and who was also a leading physician in the field diagnosed my problem from X-rays and exams.

> *"My oldest daughter and her two sisters each had a 50/50 chance of inheriting [my disease]."*

My MED diagnosis was an educated guess; back in the '60s, the doctor couldn't tell us why I got it. We knew it had been passed down from my mom, who grew up not knowing what disease she had, nor the origin. We couldn't identify any of her forebears who suffered from it; it's possible the gene mutation began with her.

The exact cause of my MED remained a mystery to me until about five years ago, when my oldest daughter, who inherited my disease, underwent genetic testing at the Hospital for Special Surgery (HSS) in New York City. She has several of my afflictions, including chronic pain. She had her hips replaced in her early 30s.

HSS gave her genetic testing for free to figure out where her disease originated. Because we share some DNA, the results didn't apply just to her but also to me.

Such testing is becoming more and more common. These days, you can spit in a tube and get your DNA data, from your ancestry to the chance you might get cancer or Alzheimer's. Or you can explore your possible genetic destiny by swabbing the inside of your cheek (like they do on cop shows). More involved testing requires taking blood or amniotic fluid, which assesses DNA before birth.

But is this kind of testing a boon or bane to our world? How would you react to knowing your DNA caused a painful disease? That is more relevant as genetic testing technology rapidly advances.

We can now know ourselves on the deepest level — the DNA that makes us who we are. Is that knowledge comforting or confounding?

MY MUTATION

According to the National Organization for Rare Diseases (NORD), MED is "estimated to occur in approximately 1 in 20,000 people in the general population."

Lucky me.

The name contains clues to how the disease works:

- "Multiple," referring to several bones and joints where it occurs

- "Epiphyseal," referring to a problem with the epiphyses, the ends of the long bones in the body like the femur (upper leg), where the problem lies

- "Dysplasia," referring to the bones and joints being displaced and deformed.

Basically, for those of us with MED, the ends of the long bones don't grow together correctly, so that the cartilage can't do its job of absorbing shock, reducing friction, and helping the joints move smoothly. Age and wear put more strain on joints, eventually causing osteoarthritis, the most common form of arthritis, which about 80% of people over age 55 get.

The genetic test my daughter took traced our MED to the COMP (cartilage oligomeric matrix protein) gene.

Just in case you want to go looking for it on the human genome, it's on the short arm of the 19th chromosome at position 19p13.11. (The human body has 23 pairs of chromosomes in a double helix shape.) COMP came into existence as part of what evolved into humanity about 750 million years ago. It causes more than half of MED cases.

My mutant COMP gene is dominant. It can be passed along by one parent — in this case, my mother to me and my brother — and me to my first daughter. The test my eldest had also showed we have recessive genes that cause skeletal issues, which both parents must have for a characteristic to show up, that can lead to skeletal deformities.

But a defective COMP gene does not mean someone will necessarily pass along MED. My oldest daughter and her two sisters each had a 50/50 chance of inheriting it. She got it, but my other children did not.

> *"Genetics is a cruel lottery."*

My eldest daughter and my brother decided not to have kids. I hope the mutation dies with us, at least for our family, but who knows? Genetics is a cruel lottery.

GENETIC TESTING IS POPULAR

Genetic testing has boomed since scientists finished mapping the human genome in 2003.

According to Global Market Insights, the worldwide market for genetic testing was $18.6 billion in 2023 and is expected to grow to $52.3 billion by 2032.

How does this translate into the number of people who've had genetic testing? The available stats are sketchy and a bit out of date. KnowYourDNA.com added up the folks who used six leading DNA testing providers (like Ancestry and 23andMe) in the US and China. It came up with 26 million in the US and an estimated 38.5 to 50 million worldwide in 2019. The current number is likely to be much higher.

According to research published in 2023, a whopping 129,624 types of genetic tests in the US and 197,779 globally were available, 90% of which were for clinical purposes rather than research.

GENETIC TESTING IN THE NEWS

The most famous genetic tester is actor Angelina Jolie, who made news when she had her breasts, ovaries, and fallopian tubes removed due to a cancer risk uncovered by a DNA examination. She has defects in the BRCA1 and BRCA2 (pronounced "brah-kuh") genes. Normally they fend off cancer, but abnormal ones increase the threat of the disease.

Jolie might not have gotten cancer. Genetics is a game of odds. By having problems with the BRCA genes, the actress's chances of illness were increased. She made the judgment (and has inspired other women) to reduce the odds by having surgery, an agonizing choice.

Genetic testing has also been in the headlines because of the Chapter 11 bankruptcy filing of the company 23andMe, which holds DNA data for about 15 million customers. In mid-2025, it agreed to be purchased by its cofounder and former CEO. The bankruptcy raises the question in critics' minds, though, about what happens if a DNA company changes hands.

The big question: Do 23andMe users trust the current and new owners not to abuse their data?

Still, genetic testing is popular. In a study included in the National Library of Medicine, "… 75% of participants were aware of genetic testing and 19% of participants had genetic testing. Ancestry testing was the most common type of testing that the participants were aware of and had received."

Interestingly, the research also reported that minorities and the poor were less likely to know about genetic testing or to have used it.

It also concluded: "Participants with a family history of cancer were more likely to be aware of cancer genetic testing than those without, and participants with a personal history of cancer were more likely to have had cancer genetic testing."

Would you want to know that your genes showed greater odds of disease? Statista reports: "As of 2022, almost half of respondents to [a US survey] said they 'would like to know a lot' if they had a genetic change that would increase their chances of getting cancer. [J]ust under 10% said they wouldn't want to know at all."

PROS AND CONS OF GENETIC TESTING

Testing is done for a variety of reasons, reports the Mayo Clinic, among them:

- To diagnose diseases like cystic fibrosis or Huntington's disease

- To predict disease

- To determine whether a person is a disease carrier

- To identify drugs that might help a condition

- For prenatal testing

- For newborn screening

- For testing before IVF.

Besides discovering you are one-quarter Irish, the primary pro of testing, according to Michigan Medicine at the University of Michigan, is insight into your health. It can reassure you and your family members that a problem gene is not present. And it could prompt preventive lifestyle changes or, like Jolie, medical intervention to reduce chances of illness.

> *"People may feel angry, depressed, anxious, or guilty about their results."*

On the con side, people often don't consider the psychological impact of genetic testing. Observes Rajani Aatre, MS, MSc, senior genetic counselor at the Frankel Cardiovascular Center on the Michigan Medicine website:

> *The science is easy to process; the emotional component is not. Let's say you find out your kid got something because you passed it down. No matter how much you intellectualize it, you can't ever discount that the feeling of responsibility or guilt won't affect you.*

I can relate. Explains an article in the federal government's MedLine Plus:

> *People may feel angry, depressed, anxious, or guilty about their results. In some cases, genetic testing creates tension within a family because the results can reveal information about other family members in addition to the person who is tested. … The test often can't determine if a person will show symptoms of a disorder, how severe the symptoms will be, or whether the disorder will progress over time. Another major limitation is the lack of treatment strategies for many genetic disorders once they are diagnosed.*

Consider: Would you want to know whether you might get a dread disease if nothing could be done about it?

Other negatives include cost. A cheap test kit might trace ancestry, but it might not help much with disease predisposition. Also, most medical genetic testing is aimed at a particular problem; it is not an assessment of your entire body. And then there is the question of privacy protection and the possibility that DNA data might be used to discriminate in employment or eligibility for obtaining health or life insurance. Legislation has not caught up with the reality of genetic technology.

TROUBLING QUESTIONS

My daughter's genetic testing raises questions, the most troubling of which is: Would I have fathered her if I knew she would live a life in chronic pain?

The answer: She is a smart, funny, and accomplished woman. I can't imagine denying her life and I can't imagine denying me her life.

> *"Could mucking with my DNA have saved me from a lifetime of pain?"*

But there is a disconnect between genetic testing's potential and the reality of what it will mean to people.

Take, for example, gene editing techniques like CRISPR: If they had that back when I was born in the late '50s, could mucking with my DNA have saved me from a lifetime of pain? Would I want that?

And: If my mom had known that I and my brother would be handicapped, would she have had us? Would my father, who could never quite get over that his sons weren't that athletic?

And more recently, would I have gambled on that 50% chance had I known my daughters might suffer? I feel immense guilt for giving my disease to my eldest. We are estranged. The reasons are complex, but I fret that part is because she blames me for her pain.

Anyone who undergoes genetic testing and discovers a problem will likely face similar thoughts. Reading DNA to assess health shouldn't be taken lightly. Understand the pluses and minuses. Research whether it is right for you and, by extension, your family.

Don't get me wrong: I am not advocating for or against genetic testing. It has helped me and my family finally solve the mystery of where our disease comes from. There is a comfort in knowing the cause of our suffering.

Pain Points

"At age 32 I had to go to the hospital ER for sudden, excruciating lower back pain from no known cause. X-rays showed that I was born with an extra vertebra which later caused scoliosis and daily pain in my right hip and lower back. Genetic testing may or may not have revealed the extra vertebra but if I knew at an earlier age … that I had an extra vertebra I would have done more exercises to strengthen my core muscles to minimize scoliosis-induced pain later in life. Then in my mid 30s, the pinky finger on my right hand started to curl down toward my palm and I could no longer move that finger. I learned that it was a genetic condition called Dupuytren's contracture. … It made me think, Do I have any other genetic anomalies? Yep. … I 'discovered' at age 75 that I almost certainly have an extra X chromosome, a condition called Klinefelter's Syndrome. … Some people, like myself, have no real family history, whether through adoption, or as in my case, both sets of grandparents were murdered and all family history was lost. Genetic testing can at least fill in many of the blanks when there is no family history or you just want, or need, to know about potential future health problems." —Tom Lang

"I can relate to a lot of this. I have an inherited cancer syndrome called MEN1 (multiple endocrine neoplasia — type 1) that is an autosomal dominant. About one in 30,000 people have it. I gave it to my oldest; two of my kids tested negative, and our youngest three we haven't tested at this point. It's a grieving process at first, or at least it was for me. However, I've found peace in simply doing the best I can with self-care." —Lindy Vogel

"I had genetic testing done two years ago for cancer. I had stage 1 ovarian cancer in my 40s. I have two daughters and four biological granddaughters, so it was important to know. It was horribly expensive. It wiped out my HSA savings. But, I don't have the gene, which is helpful for my offspring to know." —Lori Stratton

Pain Points are comments on this essay as it appeared originally on Medium.com. They are solely the opinions of the commentators and do not necessarily reflect the views of the book author or publisher.

Pain Becomes His Profession

*A pain sufferer and "metagerontologist" helps
others navigate our maddening healthcare system*

Jacob Kendall was taking a video class for his online master of divinity degree when he ran into an issue.

The course professor insisted that all cameras be on for the Zoom sessions so she could see whether students were engaged with class.

As someone who already held an undergraduate degree in biology, three master's degrees, and a PhD in gerontology (the study of aging), the 39-year-old Kendall had no problem paying attention, so he asked for a special accommodation.

> *"I told her I have chronic pain that gets worse when I'm standing or sitting."*

> *I told her I have chronic pain that gets worse when I'm standing or sitting, especially for a long time. I have to lie down to be comfortable and concentrate during class. I said it's distracting to me and other students for me to be on camera while lying down, so I'd like to turn it off. However, she responded, 'The policy for this course is to have your camera on for all class meetings — find a way to deal with your pain.'*

Formerly a college professor himself, Kendall wondered why the instructor had so little empathy for someone with a disability.

"I think that if you can't figure out how to keep everyone engaged, you're not a good enough teacher," he says. "Don't punish students for that."

Unfortunately, that "just-get-over-it" attitude has been too prevalent in his health history, including from healthcare providers.

"Many have told me I just have to deal with the pain," Kendall says.

It's not that easy. Kendall has a range of chronic conditions, including an extensive family history of heart disease and a bad back. He's encountered America's healthcare system hundreds of times and has seen its weaknesses.

He turned his exasperation and experience into his profession, what he's coined as a "metagerontologist, someone examining and addressing issues related to aging from multiple perspectives all at once."

A PAIR OF HEART SURGERIES PLUS BACK PAIN

Kendall lives in Fairhope, Alabama, about 45 minutes from Mobile, with his wife and two young kids.

He has had two open-heart surgeries to replace faulty aortic valves; the current one is mechanical. He is on blood thinners, needs at least yearly echocardiograms, and has various peripheral issues related to his heart disease and surgeries.

Among other health issues:

"No single health issue exists in a vacuum."

I also have chronic pain in my back, which started about 2010, not long after I started grad school. Most of it is in my lower back, primarily on the right side, which tends to feel numb. An MRI showed a degenerative disc. In addition, I have unexplained pain in my mid- to upper back. It is a mix of persistent dull pains and sharp pains, almost as if a nerve is pinched. It is worst when I'm standing, although it can also be bad when I sit down. The only guarantee for relief comes from lying down, which is what I told that professor.

Kendall is adamant that his health problems are all related.

No single health issue exists in a vacuum, no matter how much our medical system insists upon remaining inefficiently siloed. My heart disease and everything else are related to one another in some kind of way, not the least of which is that I'm on blood thinners. This isn't some metaphysical conclusion of mine; the science backs me up.

BECOMING A GERONTOLOGY GENERALIST

Kendall works in his own business as a metagerontologist, which refers to using his broad background, including his doctorate in gerontology, to inspire dialogue about a wide range of health-related topics and disciplines.

I do consultations with patients, families, and caregivers who want to learn how to squeeze more juice out of their medical care, or who have specific questions about their circumstances. I don't give medical advice — I'm not a clinician — but I do freely share my own experience as a patient. I do a lot of thought leadership, especially on LinkedIn and by being a guest on podcasts; I'm up to 35 episodes or so by this point.

Kendall consults on cardiac health ("for obvious reasons and because it's the leading killer of people worldwide"), ageism, fitness and health, nutrition, senior living, retirement, dying and death, geriatrics, chronic disease, and caregiving. He doesn't consider himself an expert in any of these areas; rather, he sees himself as an authority on building bridges across the gaps between them.

"I grew up wanting to be a true Renaissance person," Kendall says. "I much prefer to be a jack-of-all-trades rather than an expert on one. So, to sum up, I consider myself to be a patient, aging, and caregiving advocate. See? Metagerontologist."

Kendall's turning his pain and other health conditions into his business is "100% intentional." He has grown tired of the inefficiencies in medical care he's witnessed over the years, so he decided to fight back.

FIGHTING FOR BETTER HEALTHCARE

We Americans should be embarrassed about the dysfunction of healthcare, yet most people probably don't realize just how bad it is. When it comes to our ridiculous, inefficient, and maddening healthcare system, push came to shove, and I'm shoving back.

Kendall frequently speaks at conferences, meetings, and church gatherings. Although he uses metagerontologist as his primary professional identity, he changes how he refers to himself based on the audience. He may say he's a "theogerontologist" (in religious contexts), public health gerontologist, global health gerontologist, or social work gerontologist.

One of his speech topics is how to build optimized patient-provider partnerships. Over the years, he's picked up good tricks, tips, strategies, and hacks (see below), primarily through fiercely assertive self-advocacy.

"There's a reason they tell you on airplanes to put on your own oxygen mask before you help anyone else do so. My health comes first. Nothing else matters if that's not true."

Kendall gets frustrated when he sees physicians doing their jobs badly.

I'm fine with the fact that they don't know everything — they shouldn't be expected to. What I'm not fine with is physicians who fail to be curious. I think the best quality they can have, outside of their own medical expertise, can be summed up by a famous adage: 'Be curious, not judgmental.'

TEACHING ABOUT DISABILITY

Kendall sees the problems that disabled folks like him face not as individual weaknesses but as a societal breakdown.

"People don't have disability. Society creates disability."

One of his favorite things to teach when he was a social work professor was the difference between the statement "A person with a wheelchair cannot access a building because of his or her disability" and the more accurate statement "A person in a wheelchair can't access a building because that building hasn't provided means of access for persons in wheelchairs."

"Disability exists not only at the individual level, but at the institutional, population, or systemic levels. In that way, people don't have disability. Society creates disability."

Kendall is also concerned about ensuring that he and others can get the healthcare they need. He notes that the population growth of his home area of LA (Lower Alabama) and elsewhere in America means that it's sometimes difficult to get prompt appointments and access.

Example: I am on Warfarin (a blood thinner) since I have a mechanical aortic valve, and therefore have a higher-than-average risk of stroke, bleeding events, and so on. When I need urgent care, I really need it. I am not exaggerating when I say that access to timely, high-quality healthcare is a life-or-death issue for me.

LEAVE NO STONE UNTURNED

Kendall advises other sufferers to "leave no stone unturned" when it comes to getting help. He's had to push physicians, nurses, and others to get the care he requires. "Ask, ask, and ask again. Be assertive, not passive or aggressive," he says.

Kendall's strategy for squeezing the most out of the healthcare system includes some practical hacks:

Track doctors

Between all the specialists he sees, it's easy to get confused. He says you should use the calendar in your phone and put your appointment there while it's being scheduled, not later. Include time, date, address, name of the providers you'll see, what specialists they are, and additional notes.

Set up calendars

Use one calendar color for healthcare appointments, and not for anything else. Every Sunday, check appointments for the coming week. Label the alarms clearly (i.e., "take evening meds"). Hit "Snooze" rather than "Stop" until you've taken the drugs. Use a unique ringtone for your alerts.

Keep an updated list of your meds in a separate note on your phone

Record the name(s) of the meds, the dosages, when and how often you take them, and other info or questions. Review the note at least once a month to ensure it is up to date. Check it before each appointment.

Bring someone with you to appointments

This could be a family member, caregiver, or friend. This person has to know the details of your medical care so he or she can help you keep detailed notes of each appointment. Include your questions and providers' answers. Review the notes with your family member, caregiver, or friend regularly.

Sign up for providers' health portals

This is where information about your appointments will be stored. Look for forms to fill out. Monitor the health data there, such as test results. Message the physicians or nurses if you have questions or need refills.

Finally, there are also mindset strategies. For example, I work on decreasing my stress. I try not to work all the time. I usually block off at least a little time each weekday, usually in the evenings, to do an activity I enjoy, such as reading, watching a movie, playing a musical instrument, playing a board game with my wife, watching sports (especially college football — Roll Tide!), and walking in nature. I'll add that though holding my kids can tire my back, the positives of playing with them are greater. Family is one of the best antidotes to just about any problem in life.

4

Career Crash

Dashed dreams, lost purpose, and damaged finances go with job loss due to pain

The moment was minimal compared to how monumental it was.

At Panera, I sat across a table from my business partner and close friend with whom I'd started a small but successful communications and marketing firm six years earlier. Now it was all ending — at least for me.

Within seconds it was over. He passed me a check for the token amount of $1, thus buying out my interest in the company. I was moving on from a six-figure salary to an uncertain financial future. I'd abandoned one of my main purposes in life, to be an earner for my family. Worse, I had sold off a major part of my core identity.

> *"[I had] no idea what the future would bring."*

After nearly four decades of my working life, after earning a bachelor's in magazine journalism, after countless staff meetings and client presentations, after thousands of miles of air and car travel, after writing and editing millions of words, after creating dozens of media properties, after founding two companies, after forming close friendships with colleagues, after meeting my future wife on the job, my career had crashed and burned.

I was only 53, far short of the classic retirement age of 65, with no idea what the future would bring.

THE RAVAGES OF A RARE DISEASE
What happened?

I sold my half of the business because I needed to get out. I just couldn't continue to work anymore.

29

Building a Second Career in Disability

In researching this essay on how chronic pain crashes careers, I came upon a story from *Forbes* that talks about turning disabilities into second careers.

The writer interviewed two founders with chronic illness. Emily Levy is the co-founder of Mighty Well, which sells accessories to accommodate those with disabilities, and Hannah Olson started Chronically Capable, a company that "connects those with chronic illness and disabilities with flexible job opportunities at progressive companies who have greater willingness to be inclusive and make accommodations."

Of working while ill, Levy says in the article, "I've had to learn to be very transparent in my needs. I'm not afraid to tell people, sorry, today I just can't do it. ... My health really is my first job, and Mighty Well, for better or worse, will always be my second job, because if my health isn't there, I can't really function at work."

In the story, Olson advises those in chronic pain who are also job seekers to disclose their need for accommodations to prospective employers right away. "It's a lot easier than waiting six months into the job and having to have this awkwardness," she says.

You see, I was born with a rare genetic disease, causing, among other conditions, chronic pain.

I held back the disease for most of my life. As a child and teen, I rode my bike all over my hometown in the San Fernando Valley in Los Angeles. I played pick-up basketball and wrestled with my friends in the pool. I went to college at Boston University and roamed Beantown and environs. I married, fathered three daughters, and did family things like visiting Walt Disney World and vacationing at the beach. I built a career in journalism, marketing, and entrepreneurship that allowed us to buy comfortable homes, keep the bills paid, put our kids through college, and build a nest egg for retirement.

I put a lot of miles on my body. By the time I entered my 50s, it had broken down.

I'd already had four joint replacements (both hips twice), starting at age 27. A nurse who saw my chart that first time assumed the age on it was a typo, that I really must have been 72. She was shocked when she came into my room for the first time and found a young adult in bed, ready to have his hip ripped out and replaced with titanium.

Later, as I came into my sixth decade, both my feet had bent at the ankles by 45 degrees, causing me to walk on the outside edges, which doctors call supination. This was extremely painful and forced me to use a wheelchair to get around.

My whole body hurt, particularly the weight-bearing and active joints of the ankles, knees, and shoulders, which I could feel becoming unstable.

It didn't help that I was pushing 250 pounds on my 5-foot, 8-inch frame, putting extra pressure on my joints.

All this had a severe impact on how I could do my job, which involved lots of travel to work with clients around the country. And the chronic pain I dealt with messed with the concentration, communication, and creativity I needed to do it well. Thanks to this reality, I simply couldn't continue professionally.

I was forced to call it a career.

CAREER PROBLEMS FOR SUFFERERS

Other chronic pain sufferers can relate to the reality of giving up their jobs because of their conditions. Research shows chronic pain crushes careers.

For example, about three out of four of American adults who suffer from HICP (pain that not only lasts longer than the normal healing process but that interferes with sufferers' daily lives) are unemployed.

Pain is the number-one reason people miss work. The economic hit of chronic pain to America is greater than that of heart disease, cancer, and diabetes.

Those who work when in chronic pain are frequently distressed and unhappy. According to a study in the National Library of Medical Information, employees in chronic pain are:

- 64% less likely to view their job as rewarding

- 47% more likely to be subjected to threats/abuse in the workplace

- 30% more likely to report poor supervisor support

- 28% more likely to perceive discrimination in the workplace.

The same source says those with pain missed about

There are provisions of US law that provide rights for those who need help to get their jobs done. This includes, for example, arranging for remote work, which became widespread during the pandemic.

"We've learned … that an employee doesn't necessarily need to be in an office in order to be productive and that you can be working on your own hours," Olson says. "So many people were left out of the workplace simply because of the fact that they couldn't physically be in an office. This is opening up a world of opportunities for those who had been previously left out."

Olson says she's garnered great satisfaction from being an entrepreneur with chronic illness. "We talk so much about all that has been taken from us with our illness. And it's true, so much has been stripped of me, but I've also gained so much. … I wouldn't regret being chronically ill now because I've been able to learn and do so much more than I ever would've."

"I soon embarked on what I call surgerypalooza."

nine more days of work per year than respondents without pain. "Chronic pain was associated with lower vocational fulfillment and feelings of being ostracized in the workplace," the researchers concluded.

It's no leap to assert that chronic pain sufferers who work are likely vastly underemployed.

SURGERY FEST

After leaving my last job, I soon embarked on what I call my surgerypalooza.

Starting in 2012, I had twin operations to fuse my ankles and return my feet to being flat, allowing me to walk again. Over the following years, I also had both knees and both shoulders replaced.

Each recovery was excruciating and involved plenty of physical therapy and powerful opioids. Before authorities found that OxyContin was extremely addictive, I was up to three 80-milligram pills (the strongest dose available) a day. Fortunately, I never became addicted.

Toward the end of the 2010s, I added bariatric sleeve surgery to cut my stomach down to the size of a banana peel. I did it to slim down and reduce the strain on my joints. Over about six months, I lost 80 pounds.

In all, I've had eight joint replacements plus the ankle and bariatric surgery. But I still feel chronic pain from head to toe. I use a cane and a wheelchair to get out and about. Powerful medications (see chapter 7) allow me to function and maintain a decent quality of life despite all my problems.

Physically, though, I'm a wreck.

DING TO MY IDENTITY

Retiring early was a shock to my system.

During my adult life, identified first as a husband and father, my profession was a part of my core image of myself. I had dreams of writing for big-time publications like *The New Yorker* or publishing best-sellers. Being a provider and protector of my family had all to do with my economic value. My identity as a writer, editor, and entrepreneur was embedded in my personal psyche. My drive to achieve ran deep.

I was raised to be a grade grubber. My parents paid my brother and me for A's and academic accomplishments. I won a full tuition scholarship to Boston University and was nominated for a Rhodes Scholarship. After college, I joined a hot startup led by a charismatic founder who produced magazines and other media for schools, universities, businesses, and healthcare offices. I carried on from there to work for other firms and, eventually, start a couple of companies, including the one I sold for pennies just to get out.

I say this not to brag but to show the depth of my praise-junkie depravity. Those glory days are long gone, leaving a part of me feeling empty.

My genetic disease truncated me. I might have been taller. I might have been stronger. I might have reached my "gifted" potential.

As Marlon Brando says in *On the Waterfront*, "I coulda been a contender. I coulda been somebody."

Perhaps all this was just wishful thinking, of course. I'll never know what I could have become as a person and a professional had I not had my disease.

It's hard, though, not to think about what might have been.

FINANCIAL WOES AND BLOWS

Chronic pain stole my 50s, some of my prime earning years.

Fortunately, my wife worked as a freelance writer for such publications as *National Geographic Traveler*. I felt guilty, though, for shifting the primary breadwinning from me to her, a blow to my male ego. I was never a fan of husband-works-wife-stays-at-home thinking. I did, however, feel a huge responsibility to provide for my family. It was difficult to let that attitude go.

Savvily, I had kept paying for disability insurance from that first job for the charismatic founder out of college. With the help of the company that held the policy, I also applied for Social Security Disability Insurance (SSDI) right away and was accepted the first try, something I'm told is rare. Because I had been a relatively high earner, it paid a few thousand dollars a month, which saved our financial life.

Before I qualified for regular Social Security at my full retirement age, I lived "on the dole" for more than a decade.

The constant financial worries ground on us. Even though we had already put our daughters through college, my forced retirement made it difficult to keep our quality of life. I fretted endlessly about where the money would come from.

During those years, I had recurring dreams of being back at work, trying to please the company founder, and failing. Each time, I couldn't do the job due to my chronic condition and would awake terrified of being unemployed.

LOSS OF PURPOSE

And then there was the sense of purposelessness, something many retirees, forced or not, experience.

My surgeries and recoveries took up a lot of time with doctors' visits, hospital stays, and physical therapy appointments. But that still leaves a ton of time to ponder life and think about what my career and life amounted to. Not to get too existential, but reflection raised questions of what legacy I'd leave. Was being a husband, father, and, eventually, grandfather enough? The problem was both philosophical and practical: What was I to do with myself in retirement?

To keep my hand in writing and editing, I authored an unpublished (and likely unpublishable) 400,000-word novel about a serial killer that murders bad parents. I did this between pangs of pain as I sat in the welcome comfort of my La-Z-Boy. I made no money, of course. I was in it as a creative pastime.

> *"[Making money] wasn't the point."*

Then, in 2021, my middle daughter gave me a present for my birthday: a $50 Amazon gift card. I turned this into a keyboard for my iPad. It was a small change, but it unleashed my ability to write with my disability easily versus the difficulty of using a relatively bulky laptop.

Something reawakened in me.

I got the idea of creating a book that captured what I'd learned during my decades as a communicator. With the help of some former colleagues, I self-published *Seven Cs: The Elements of Effective Writing* on Amazon in 2022.

I didn't expect to, and haven't, made much money from that, but doing so wasn't the point. It was the satisfaction of showing myself that I could still pull off complicated publishing projects.

Some of the confidence I'd lost when my career crashed was reborn. I felt pride in the craftsmanship the book took. It not only passed the time and gave me a reason to get up in the morning, but it was something I could do despite my handicap.

I've continued to pursue writing as a mostly unpaid hobby. I've created essays about chronic pain and the feelings it brings, which have turned into this book. If any money comes from this, it will be a bonus.

My point, though, is that after a decade of *meh*, I've found purpose, identity, and a bit of financial hope. And though my experience is unique to my situation, it shows other sufferers that chronic pain need not permanently blow up their lives and livelihoods.

ADVICE FOR FELLOW SUFFERERS

I urge my fellow chronic pain sufferers to explore your creativity, passions, and interests despite the limitations of having debilitating disabilities.

I understand that it is hard to muster the energy to do something like writing when you feel terrible because of chronic conditions. Believe me, I know the feeling. But the truth is, writing heals (see chapter 34).

On bad days when my pain flares, I just can't produce anything. I don't beat myself up, though. I chalk it up to another reality of living with my genetic disease. But on other days, I feel better and can put in a couple of hours a day creating essays like this one.

Inspirational stories of entrepreneurs who deal with chronic pain (see sidebar) reinforce my quest to pursue my own creative passions and find greater fulfillment in retirement.

Wish me luck with my second act.

Pain Points

"My traumatic head and spine injury crippled me from the workplace. … The brain injury [also] caused epilepsy and between the two, I couldn't focus or complete simple tasks for almost two years. I missed my window by the time it dawned on me. Now, I feel lucky to have re-careered into a creative field and to be earning. But I couldn't survive on my current income, and spine injuries are progressive, so I guess it's time for another surgery. It really does weigh on the ego. Sad. This was done to me." —Tabitha Warren

"I was 53, too, when I got a chronic illness. It eroded my self-worth for a while particularly because it impacted my reputation in my career. I realized I had made the mistake of entwining my identity with my work. … I found solace and mental healing through creativity (mainly through writing)." —Kay Flanagan

"'Writing heals.' I will continue repeating it to myself." —Stephany Thomann

Pain Points are comments on this essay as it appeared originally on Medium.com. They are solely the opinions of the commentators and do not necessarily reflect the views of the book author or publisher.

5

$2 Million Lost

*The bill for pain to US society and sufferers is
more than $722 billion a year*

I spent the last decade or so getting joints ripped out of my body and replaced by metal, ceramics, and plastic.

As you can imagine, I experienced a whole lot of pain, not all of it physical. There has been plenty of financial distress, too, given all the cash that I've laid out for operations, treatments, physical therapy, and other healthcare.

I am not alone. Millions of American adults and children have chronic pain and it costs them and our society hundreds of billions of dollars. Fortunately, I have a simple prescription for cutting that cost.

"I calculated what the total cost [of pain] has been to me."

HOW MUCH CHRONIC PAIN HAS COST ME

As an example of the personal price of pain, in early 2025 I calculated what the total cost has been to me. I'm lucky that I had medical insurance that paid for most of my care, but yearly I was responsible for thousands of dollars out of pocket for all my surgeries, not to mention scores of doctors' visit copays.

I've had various procedures, from epidurals to cortisone shots, each with a price. I've paid for medications to ease my pain, including fentanyl patches. I fund physical therapy in a swimming pool twice a week. And I've invested in everything from a metal knee brace to a bone stimulator (a machine that supposedly causes bone to grow after an injury or operation) to the unreimbursed wheelchair I use to get around.

My sloppy accounting shows that I spend an average of $6,400 annually for healthcare (not including health insurance premiums). Extend that figure back

Prescription to Cut Chronic Pain Costs

As a sufferer who's borne the burden of paying for chronic pain, I have a simple prescription for easing the cost to individuals and society: Cut pain itself.

There are easy, relatively affordable ways to ease suffering:

Improve pain education
Teach the entire healthcare community about pain science by adding required attendance at classes in medical, nursing, physical therapy, and chiropractic schools as well as continuing medical education (CME) programs.

Invest in pain research
Rather than spending billions just on drugs and devices, focus instead on sufferers' experience of pain, which is both physical and mental. Develop therapies that address the body and soul.

Increase public awareness of pain
Most people don't think about chronic pain until they're in it. Publicize pain as a serious public health problem, one worthy of attention even when there are other illnesses to worry about.

35 years, during which I suffered the majority of enduring hurt, and that's a total of $224,000. Not exactly chump change.

And that doesn't count the price I've paid in unrealized wages. I wrote in the last chapter about how chronic pain crashed my career and forced me to retire. It wiped out my prime earning years of my 50s through retirement age.

If I'd continued to earn the salary I had before retirement, those years would be worth about another $1.5 million if I never received another raise or benefited from income inflation. And, of course, I didn't put away more cash for retirement in a company 401(k) that might have grown with the booming stock market. I estimate the employment opportunity cost was $1.75 million in all.

So, throw in the $224,000 for medical care and call the price of pain to me a conservative $2 million in direct and indirect money I could have used for other things — a dream house? a shiny new car? travel around the world? — had I not had chronic pain and associated problems.

Don't get me wrong: I'm not whining about all the money I've lost. I'm simply pointing out how costly chronic pain can be. Everyone has his or her own cross to bear and economic consequences come with it.

CHRONIC PAIN IS EXPENSIVE

The US itself pays a high price for pain.

A study published in 2025 put the cost of pain to American society in 2021 at $722.8 billion, which includes $530.6 billion in medical care and $192.2 billion in lost work productivity.

That means each individual with chronic pain paid

$8,068 in yearly medical expenses and $2,923 in lost productivity, or about $11,000 per person, as compared to someone without enduring hurt. My accounting of the personal price of pain is much less than this, so I'm probably underestimating what I've lost.

It's difficult for people in the worst chronic pain to make the money to pay the price of pain. Consider that 83% of people with high impact chronic pain (HICP), that which interferes with activities of daily life, are unemployed.

"Each individual ... paid $8,068 in yearly medical expenses and $2,923 in lost productivity, or about $11,000 per person."

And for those who do work, pain has an impact on personal productivity. On average, people with severe pain miss between five and six more workdays a year. It's no big leap to conclude that people with chronic pain tend to be poorer than peers without hurt.

TALLYING THE TRUE PRICE OF PAIN

The bottom line: Chronic pain costs. Lots. It's enormously expensive for individuals and society, both through direct payments and indirect ones, such as the increasing price of medical insurance.

The best way to cut the cost of pain, though, is to cut pain itself. Reduce the quantity and quality of people's suffering and it will become less expensive for individuals and society.

Compared to cancer, heart disease, or diabetes, there has been little focus by healthcare policymakers on solving the problem of pain. As it goes unaddressed, pain and suffering add up.

We all pay for pain, for example, in disbursements for Social Security disability, Medicare, and Medicaid. Employers pay in lost productivity and days missed on the job. The healthcare system spends billions trying to identify and treat pain, often inefficiently and ineffectively.

Until we recognize the true cost of pain — the agony and desperation of sufferers — the economic damage will only continue.

See the sidebar for my prescription for cutting the cost of pain. The final part of it is simple, though: Increase compassion among physicians, policymakers, and the public.

To cut the cost of pain, we must come together to care more, give more comfort, and express more concern.

That last part isn't expensive.

All it costs is some kindness.

Pain Points

"I have some very kind providers and yet I can sense when they're out of options as invariably I end up being told I just have to think about my pain differently. How about we work a little harder to sort out why I'm in pain enough to have lost so many of the activities I enjoy? Isn't there something else available to ease this constant discomfort? Many times, I've tried something new and thought, *Okay this time it will be different.* And once again, I'm back where I started. Better and deeper education in pain management would benefit us all." —Kate Fallon

"I am a Dutch national living in Luxembourg. Four months ago I had a hip replacement, had to stay in hospital longer than normal, five days, due to a fever which the doctors would not send me home with. I have a state health insurance which costs me about €100 per month and on top of that I paid €153 myself. ... Is it not the responsibility of our governments to provide healthcare and not create circumstances for insurance companies to become filthy rich?" —Big Benny

"Without taking anything away from your current experience — as I understand you can't do much about being born with a genetic disease like MED — let's take the lens deeper, and more multigenerational. What are we doing to the ecosystems (of which we are a part) that is messing with our genetics? What are we doing to our food supply and our nervous systems? What are we doing in society that causes hormonal disruptions? Where is this pain coming from? ... [I]f we keep working downstream of the pain, instead of swimming upstream to find its abundant and growing headwaters, we're going to keep chasing our tails." —Kaia Maeve Tingley

Pain Points are comments on this essay as it appeared originally on Medium.com. They are solely the opinion of the commentators and do not necessarily reflect the views of the book author or publisher.

6

Struggling With Dis-ease

*Those of us with chronic pain contend
with constant stress*

Sometimes my wife asks me, "How ya doin'?"

"I'm fine," I lie.

After nearly 40 years of marriage, we can read each other's body language. She knows me well enough to tell when something is wrong. I understand that she worries about me, but I don't want to burden her yet again with my true feelings.

Most of the time, I am not fine.

My chronic pain is a relentless opponent, an all-consuming ache from head to toe, punctuated by severe stabs in spots like the lower back, hands, and neck. My body is a mass of inflammation because of my rare genetic disease.

> *"My chronic pain is a relentless opponent."*

Among other emotions, my disease causes dis-ease. The derivation of the former, as in an illness, comes from the 14th-century French combination of *des*, "without, away," and *aise*, "ease," so it literally meant "without ease."

That's an apt definition of what I feel most of the time: a lack of ease, a dis-ease.

SEDENTARY LIFESTYLE

I envy able-bodied people who go through life seemingly free of anxiety about their movements, like climbing stairs, walking the dog, or parking far away from a movie theater entrance. These people don't have to think about whether their next move will be painful.

In contrast, I spend a lot of time sitting in my La-Z-Boy, the only place I feel comfortable, but still the aches and pains lurk. In lighter moments, I imagine launching a lifestyle brand called: "Sedentary: For Those Who Hurt Too Much to Move."

I hurt, but my discomfort goes beyond body pain to psychological distress. The constant worry makes it hard to truly enjoy life. I spend so much time and energy enduring the physical sensations and considering how to mitigate them that I often cannot think straight. I can't turn it off. It's an irritating, deeply frustrating buzz in my body.

I live in a state of stress and anxiety. For me, it's like having persistent tinnitus, also called ringing of the ears. It's a constant hum of hurt. My chronic pain is a continuing companion messing with my mind.

THE SCIENCE OF DIS-EASE

There's science behind these feelings.

Brian Distelberg, PhD, MA, and Director of the Behavioral Health Institute at Loma Linda University Health, explains:

> When someone experiences pain, the body releases anxiety and stress hormones. This can come in handy if a person is injured or in a situation where they need to get out. However, when we look at an individual who is constantly experiencing pain, then the body is also constantly producing these toxic hormones as well. Stress isn't an intangible thing — it's a damaging chemical to the body when prolonged.

This damage interferes with my life. For example, my body and mind are perpetually on point. My jaw constantly clenches, bracing for the pain. My muscles are always taut, ready to spring into action, even when I'm not moving. My stomach and GI tract roil with fear about what's to come — in the short term, with the next step, and in the long term, with how much worse I'll be as I age.

My brain is on guard all the time, causing me to wince when nerves send it pain signals. I get nightly headaches behind my forehead. I imagine that's all due to those stress hormones flowing through me, heightening my overactive Spidey-sense.

Science calls this hypervigilance, which can increase chronic pain.

FIGHT, FLIGHT, FREEZE

In short, I am in a perpetual state of fight, flight, or freeze — an ancient instinct that saved humans from threats such as lions, tigers, and bears. When I walk with my cane, I look down for hazards, calculating my next step, and fretting that taking it will sting.

You can miss a lot of life when you're always looking down.

"I am in a perpetual state of fight, flight, or freeze."

I tell myself to relax, which is kind of an oxymoron because you can't force yourself into a state of bliss. I can't just convince myself to take it easy, despite years of therapy focused on reframing my thinking. I've tried meditation and deliberate breathing to no avail; the anxiety prevents me from quieting my mind.

It's like anticipating a jump scare in a *Halloween* movie: Pain stalks me like Michael Myers. On the worst days, which thankfully don't happen often, this fear leads to depression, hopelessness, and despair.

THE IMPACT OF DIS-EASE

Battling pain means that I'm sometimes not as present for my family as I'd like to be.

When my wife tells me about her day shuttling our toddler granddaughter around town, I try to pay close attention, but am many times dragged away by my painful body and preoccupied mind. I spend so much physical and mental energy enduring the pain that I sometimes have little left over for anything else. She loves me and I love her, but my distraction creates distance between us.

I apologize to her and the rest of my family for not always being there for them.

The thing besides health and happiness for my family that I want most in life: peace of mind.

The thing I cannot ever have because of my dis-ease: peace of mind.

Don't worry. I'm fine.

PAIN PROFILE

Craving Relief

*A newly graduated graphic artist hates to think
about living the rest of her life in pain*

All Katie Schweiger wanted to do was eat a chicken sandwich with no chewing problems or chronic pain.

The 25-year-old Minneapolis native had been denied that pleasure for years because of issues with her temporomandibular joint (TMJ), which connects the jawbone to the skull. She says:

> My pain is all over my body but is worse in the jaw. It's mostly all achy all day every day, but I get random stabbing pain that lasts for about a minute at a time. I never know when it will strike. Each day, it's a different spot and type of pain that will be my face for the day.

"My knees, ankles, and hips are like the tin man's in Wizard of Oz. *"*

The winters in Minnesota are a particular challenge. "In the cold, my body feels frozen," Schweiger explains. "My knees, ankles, and hips are like the tin man's in *Wizard of Oz*."

Schweiger also suffers from chronic fatigue that made it difficult to keep up her studies at the University of Minnesota-Twin Cities. Despite her pain and exhaustion, she graduated in May 2025. She then helped design this book.

CHRONIC PAIN STARTED EARLY

At age 11, Schweiger was diagnosed with an overbite. Her orthodontist recommended a Herbst appliance in addition to braces and rubber bands to correct the problem. Though the design of Herbst appliances might vary, most are cemented on the upper molars and lower molars (or lower bicuspids) with metal arms attached from the upper to lower part of the appliance.

The orthodontist added that young Schweiger could expect the elaborate device, braces, and rubber bands to take up to three years to give her a normal bite.

"But it took much longer than expected because the rubber bands weren't doing what they were supposed to," Schweiger says. "I needed even thicker ones to keep my bite where it was supposed to be."

By 2015, four years later, she still had the braces and had developed chronic pain in her jaw and face muscles from all the hardware and effort to keep her bite corrected, which, unfortunately, didn't solve the problem.

> *"What a relief to finally see my teeth after almost six years!"*

"That's when my orthodontist had a very serious talk with me and my mom about jaw surgery," Schweiger says. "And that was a moment that I will never forget. That was the one thing that we were trying so hard to avoid."

A PAIR OF PAINFUL OPERATIONS

Schweiger says that during high school she was a theater kid, but her pain and fatigue interfered with her performances:

> *Obviously, I wanted to be there, but physically my body couldn't handle doing theater every day after school. During the beginning of my junior year, we did* The Wiz *and all these different dance numbers. Doing more than one or two each day just really wore me out.*

About that same time, when she was 17, Schweiger had the first of two operations by an oral and maxillofacial surgeon to correct her overbite and reduce her pain. First, he did lower jaw surgery and a genioplasty (surgery that realigns the chin by cutting and moving part of the chin bone) to bring her chin forward.

> *The recovery was horrible, but my bite was perfect. Six months later the braces came off and my oral surgeon cleared me — saying no more follow-up appointments. What a relief to finally see my teeth after almost six years!*

Or so she thought. The next year, Schweiger's overbite returned, accompanied by "an inability to chew correctly and really bad jaw pain."

A second operation four years later in 2022 seemed to be a success, but her jaw pain once again returned, especially near her ears. Her surgeon figured that her jaw muscles were being strained, so he prescribed muscle relaxers, which didn't help. He then recommended Schweiger see a physical therapist.

The PT explained in understandable ways what was happening and taught me what was going on in the brain to cause my pain. We figured out what helped and what didn't. He assigned me to write about what pain means to me. It was one of the most therapeutic things I've ever done."

DETERMINED TO GET ANSWERS

In the essay, Schweiger wrote about what it's like to be a young person in chronic pain:

To me, pain can get so frustrating and debilitating. I don't get to do or eat normal things with my friends because my face hurts too much — but I have too much energy to sleep. … Sometimes my pain doesn't 'turn off' … and then I wake up in the middle of the night and … getting back to sleep takes forever because my face hurts. … Sometimes it feels like the pain from my jaw [goes] through my entire body.

"When my PT read the essay," Schweiger says, "we went over every concern I had. We highlighted, we talked, I cried. Typing everything was such a needed release of my feelings."

She dreads the idea that she may need more operations.

Going through surgery twice isn't fun, and thinking about going through it again makes me want to cry. It takes the pain and stress to a whole new level, making my clenching worse.

Between 2022 and 2024, Schweiger had well over 100 appointments with doctors, pain specialists, an orthodontist, and an oral surgeon, all looking to help her figure out the cause of her pain, fatigue, and other symptoms.

Unfortunately, she doesn't yet have a satisfactory diagnosis. One doctor concluded she has fibromyalgia, but she truly doesn't believe that is what is causing so much pain and fatigue. It has been an ongoing mystery that her providers, especially her primary care doctor, want to solve.

She hasn't given up on a cure, but the thought of living in pain for the rest of her life is daunting.

I do know it is a possibility. I would love a cure, but I really just want to know what is going on. I will be searching for answers with doctors and researching on my own. I am determined to get answers.

LIFE-CHANGING PAIN

Chronic pain changed Schweiger's life in so many ways — good and bad.

I'll start with the bad. When I was in college, I didn't have the energy to work on projects over the weekends. I had to lie down or nap a lot, then I'd work harder during the week on my design work.

The positive part of dealing with her pain is that she developed an interest in medical graphic design. All the appointments she's had in the past year and a half and the amount of time spent in orthodontics and with the oral surgeon led her to write her thesis on helpful, proper patient education. Her dream is to use her skills to redesign the experience that pain sufferers like her endure daily.

My final project was a surgery recovery kit. The pamphlets and brochures, handouts, readings, and more showed me how to create patient education that actually makes sense for patients, their caregivers, and the general public.

As part of her portfolio, Schweiger reworked the problematic pain scale (see chapter 21) used by the medical community into a scale that makes more sense to her. The traditional scale rates pain from 0 (no pain) to 10 (worst pain imaginable) but doesn't capture the real experience she had.

Her redesign was inspired by other alternative pain scales Schweiger saw online and merely part of a student project, but she someday hopes she can use her experience and expertise to improve healthcare communications for people like her.

ADVICE FOR OTHER SUFFERERS

Some advice I would give to other pain sufferers is to get a really comfy pillow for your head, then get more pillows — the cheap ones or the old ones are fine — but enough to surround your body like a bird's nest. You need to comfort yourself.

And she recommends snuggle therapy.

My cat's purr is so calming and reminds me that it is okay to rest when I need to. My grandparents' dog also puts a smile on my face. And he is a snuggle-bug too.

Schweiger felt dismissed by a rheumatologist she saw, who diagnosed her with fibromyalgia but ignored her jaw pain.

He had a really poor bedside manner, and just said, 'Well, this is it. This is the only possibility it could be,' rather than 'I think there could be something else.'

I was very frustrated. Thankfully, my mom was with me because I definitely cried in the appointment, especially because we kept mentioning my jaw and he ignored that part. My mom and I were both very angry and frustrated especially because it had taken four months to get to see this doctor.

Still, Schweiger also advises her fellow sufferers to persist in their quest for solutions. "It is so hard not getting answers, and it would be so easy to give up. Don't!"

She also suggests finding a group of friends who are supportive.

It's hard to make friends as a young adult. Find people who really understand what you are going through, who can be caring and compassionate and who check up on you.

Schweiger tries not to think much about how it will be if she must live the rest of her life in chronic pain. She'd like to get a firm diagnosis for how she feels. She is overwhelmed when she thinks, *Wow. I'm only in my 20s and I've got this big thing to deal with.*

> "My cat's purr is so calming and reminds me that it is okay to rest when I need to."

Even if there's no cure or treatment for what I have, I would at least like to know it's something besides fibromyalgia. Just for my own sanity, because it's driving me crazy not being able to research my condition beyond that.

CRAVING THAT CHICKEN SANDWICH

And what about that chicken sandwich she wanted so badly?

Yes. Yes. So, after the first surgery, I really wanted a Jimmy John's sandwich. I craved that the whole recovery time. Then after the second surgery and getting the all-clear to chew again, all I wanted was a chicken sandwich. I went to Chick-fil-A. Their lemonade is my favorite. I drove home and took a picture with the sandwich in front of my face to share with all my friends about how excited I was.

And did it live up to her expectations?

"Oh, yeah. It was *delicious*."

7

28 Pills a Day Plus Fentanyl

Am I a victim of polypharmacy? Are you?

When I take my pills in the morning, it feels as though I'm swallowing an entire pharmacy.

Like millions of Americans, I take multiple prescription drugs, over-the counter (OTC) medications, and supplements.

As of this writing, here's what I start the day with:

- 2 blood-red capsules for depression

- 1 rectangular white pill for anxiety

- 2 yellow "horse pill" multivitamins to get the nutrients I need

- 1 purple-and-gray capsule for acid reflux

- 1 pink pill for allergies

- 2 round brown pills for pain

- 1 oblong white pill, also for pain

- 1 round white pill, again for pain.

> *"That's 11 pills down my throat before I've had my morning Diet Coke."*

That's 11 pills down my throat before I've had my morning Diet Coke. Then, throughout the day and at bedtime, I take 17 more.

Add everything up and I take 28 pills a day and use a fentanyl patch, the latter for pain.

How to Prevent Inappropriate Polypharmacy

Again, I am not a doctor, but I have some general advice from a patient's perspective for those concerned about inappropriate polypharmacy for themselves or a loved one:

Don't assume all polypharmacy is wrong
You may need all the drugs you take and your physicians may have good reasons for prescribing them. Some even argue for "rational polypharmacy," which means getting beyond the knee-jerk assumption that many drugs equals unacceptable danger and carefully weighing the good and bad effects of a mixture of medications.

Inform all your doctors about all the medicines and supplements you are taking
This includes OTC ones as well as those you get from online and stand-alone vitamin and supplement stores. Although primary care physicians should be responsible for monitoring our overall health, they can't if they don't have the full picture.

Specialists are organized into silos based on body parts — neurologists are responsible for the brain; ENT docs for ear, nose, and throat; dermatologists for skin; and so on. It's easy to get multiple specialists prescribing different

HOLY POLYPHARMACY

There's a name for the mess of medication I use: polypharmacy.

It is most often defined as taking five or more drugs a day; I clock in at 12 different medications (healthcare researchers call 10 or more "excessive polypharmacy"). I've also seen polypharmacy defined as using two or more medications for the same condition, which I also do.

Slowly, inexorably over the decades, my doctors added medications to address my health problems, including not just my chronic pain but also depression, anxiety, acid reflux, insomnia, low thyroid, and allergies.

I can't remember just when what doctor added what drug, which is part of the problem. Over time, the number of medications built up.

What's so bad about that?

The problem comes with "inappropriate polypharmacy," when prescribing gets out of control and momentum keeps the drugs coming each month, without anyone, including me, paying much attention to whether they might no longer be effective or needed. Worse yet, the medications might interact with each other in dangerous, even deadly, ways.

The people in the US at risk of polypharmacy include the 56 million or so adults aged 65 or older (like me) and the 60 or so million who suffer from chronic pain (like me).

Am I a victim of improper polypharmacy? Are you?

POLYPHARMACY IS WIDESPREAD

Multiple prescriptions are common. According to the National Poll on Healthy Aging, 82% of adults aged 50 to 80 take a prescription in a typical week. About three in 10 use five or more. (That's me, again.)

As for OTC medications, 60% of seniors use at least one during a typical week, with 11% taking three or more. And supplements — such as vitamins, minerals, or herbal remedies — are widespread; 78% of older adults take one or more.

Seniors are at most risk of polypharmacy, with older women particularly vulnerable because they tend to begin to take multiple drugs younger and they make up the largest swath of more mature people. Lower socioeconomic class, and therefore poorer health, also can correlate to polypharmacy. Anyone, though— old, young, rich, poor — can fall victim.

I am not an older woman or lower economic class, but I am a chronic pain sufferer. "Polypharmacy is the rule rather than the exception among persons living with chronic pain," concluded one study included in the National Library of Medicine.

It reported polypharmacy among 71.4% of chronic pain patients, who used an average of six medications. Excessive polypharmacy (using 10 or more drugs) happened to about one-quarter of sufferers.

The chances of polypharmacy among chronic pain sufferers are increased by having other medical conditions. More than 70% experience "comorbidities," which simply means they have one or more other health problems in addition to pain, according to a study reported in the journal *Plos One*.

Other research found an even higher rate of other problems, according to a 2025 survey of sufferers by the U.S. Pain Foundation:

Respondents reported an average of 10 distinct diagnoses per person. Conditions like back pain

drugs and not knowing what the others are doing. When doctors (or more likely, nurses) ask what medications you take, be sure to include everything. It's smart to hand them a typed, dated list with dosages and frequency.

Keep the list on your phone of the names and dosages of the drugs you take. Update it.
Particularly if you take several, it's not always easy to remember them all. Be sure to type the correct spellings as some drug names are similar to others.

If you have an iPhone, Apple has included an app — simply called, in Apple minimalist tradition, "Health" — that can track your medications, including any drug interactions or those with alcohol, cannabis, and tobacco. In the app, go to Medications under the Browse menu to enter what you take. There are multiple ways to enter your drugs, including scanning the pill bottles with your phone's camera. It is a bit time-consuming to get all the info in, but I can see Health becoming a significant tool in helping me keep all my drugs straight.

If possible, buy all your prescriptions from one pharmacy
Pharmacists are an underused resource. Even though they seem busier than ever, ask yours to go through your

prescriptions and look for harmful interactions. They have access to medical apps designed for this very task.

As an alternative, WebMD has a drug interaction checker. Medscape offers another. I checked some of my meds and what I found was scary: there were several serious interactions. But prescribing drugs is a risk/benefit business. Doctors balance whether a particular medication will help more than harm. If you are concerned about interactions you find, talk about it with your physicians.

Tell a trusted friend and/or family member about the medications you take
We are all sensitive to our privacy, but close confidants can help make sure you are taking drugs as prescribed. They may also spot negative side effects happening to you that you may not notice yourself.

Follow directions
Read the instructions and warnings that come with your prescriptions. Don't play doctor and decide to take more or less than you should. If you are confused about what to take or how, talk with your doctor or pharmacist (or both).

Speak up!
Communication is the key to managing medication. If you are taking multiple drugs, talk with your doc about

(64%), arthritis (53%), neuropathic or nerve pain (48%), osteoarthritis (42%), and fibromyalgia (37%) were among the most reported."

THE PROBLEM WITH POLYPHARMACY

At its worst, a myriad of medications can cause further injury or disease, sometimes with deadly consequences.

WebMD explains:

This happens because some medications mix poorly with other medicines in your body. Experts call this a drug interaction. There are several issues that can happen if you take too many medications. Drug interactions can lead to memory issues; falls and broken bones; kidney failure; liver failure; hospitalization; a higher risk of death.

Yikes!

Further, polypharmacy may make it hard for patients to recall exactly what medications to take and when. And it may be a hassle because they have to go to doctors and pharmacies frequently. It gets expensive because of copays and other fees.

Polypharmacy can also lead to what's called "prescribing cascades." Doctors prescribe medications, which all can cause adverse side effects. Physicians then prescribe more medicine to treat the side effects of the first drugs, which leads to more medications for more side effects and so on. Things can get out of control quickly.

Sometimes polypharmacy results in harm. Doctors are human and they make mistakes.

Take the case of singer-songwriter Kris Kristofferson, who died in September 2024. Doctors diagnosed him with Alzheimer's and depression and prescribed the appropriate drugs. Still, he declined and had trouble remembering what was happening from moment to moment.

Finally, someone stepped up and found that he actually had Lyme disease. He got off the previous drugs and, prior to his passing, his wife told *Today*:

> *He was taking all these medications for things he doesn't have, and they all have side effects. All of a sudden, he was back. Some days he's perfectly normal and it's easy to forget that he is even battling anything.*

Polypharmacy based on wrong diagnoses nearly ruined the end of Kristofferson's life.

(Disclaimer: This is a good time to again point out that I am not a doctor or other healthcare provider. Do not stop or start any drugs based on what I've said here or elsewhere. Always consult a qualified physician before beginning or ending any treatment.)

POLYPHARMACY AND ME

It's tough to tell whether I am a victim of inappropriate polypharmacy. Many times, I wonder if I am using drugs I don't really need. Are they doing the job they were supposed to do? Am I in danger?

So far, I haven't had any discernible problems, but I fret that the cocktail of drugs I use is subtly affecting me with unclear side effects.

For example, I tend to get sleepy and some of the drugs I take have that side effect. I also itch a lot and get scratchiness in my left eye. I ask myself if that's because of the drugs I'm taking or a new allergy.

I change my fentanyl patch every three days and sometimes I feel jumpy and anxious on a patch change day. My GI tract and bowels tend to roil on those days. Is it because my body needs a fresh dose of the opioid?

"deprescribing." It may be scary to question whether a drug is truly needed because of the psychological and physical dependency patients tend to develop. It's better, though, to face possible problems and fend them off before they become dangerous.

My final piece of advice: Be a vigilant consumer, not a passive patient.

My sinuses are perpetually clogged, and I have phlegm in my throat. Are my medications causing that or is my head just good at generating boogers?

Gross. Enough complaining.

I can't say any one of these symptoms is due to medication overuse.

As a senior and chronic pain sufferer, I worry that the medicines I take are dangerous, but, honestly, I also feel trapped in my drug routine. I am anxious that if I cut down or stop using my many medications, I'll throw off the delicate chemical balance that keeps me functioning. Even though I often feel like crap, it's hard to know whether that's from my underlying conditions or the supposed cures.

I've raised this with my primary care physician, of course. Though he doesn't see any direct danger from all the stuff I'm taking, he's agreed to help me wean off some of the medications gradually.

The whole thing is trial and error, one drug at a time, and see what happens. I worry about the error part and the pain and suffering it might bring.

I'm going to give cutting down on the 28 pills a go, though.

The truth is that it is often up to us patients to question whether polypharmacy is improper or not.

Pain Points

"It is sad to say humankind lives with pills now." —Health Matterof

"I take numerous pills a day for various conditions but only one is an opiate. I feel that all of these medications are helpful to my conditions because my quality of life was horrible and since I've been on this regimen I feel like a different person. I can walk and move, do laundry, and drive again. I'm not able to do anything for hours and I get tired quickly, but I can get things accomplished when before the meds I was a slug. I thank God for my doctor and the combination of medications she was smart enough to prescribe to give my life back to me." —Debra

"I had a pacemaker ... [M]y heart issues created a cascade of new prescriptions. I've gone over each one with my doctor — I've had her for 10 years and trust her — still, like you, I don't know what is cause and effect. I did have two round yellow ones and found I had mixed them up by sight alone, so she changed the prescription of one." —Sharon Johnson

"Most of my prescriptions are psychiatric in nature — mostly due to suffering from severe trauma in the 1990s before psychiatrists knew about alternatives. My [current] psychiatrist says, 'We all had our heads up our asses.'" —Tracey Chester

Pain Points are comments on this essay as it appeared originally on Medium.com. They are solely the opinions of the commentators and do not necessarily reflect the views of the book author or publisher.

8

The Grip of 'Painsomnia'

*Nighttime is a nightmare for me, but
there are steps to save my sleep*

My earliest memory of sleeplessness is from my boyhood.

On several late nights when I was in my early teenage years, I'd try, but fail, to sleep in my bedroom at the back of the family home in the Los Angeles suburbs. Then I heard the rumble of my father's Mercedes coming up the alley.

In the '60s and '70s, he worked as an attorney for a phone company. These were the days when corporate life meant *Mad Men* style two-martini lunches and happy hours with buddies after work. I worried about him when he was out late drinking, the start of a lifetime of nights filled with anxiety and hypervigilance instead of slumber.

> *"I have never shaken the dread I feel as I try to fall sleep."*

As soon as I heard his car, I'd run out of the house to our detached two-car garage. In the dark of the night, I'd arrive just as Dad was pulling up to the garage door. By the light of his headlights, I'd unlock it and hoist it up toward the roof, clearing the way for the car to enter. My father would pull in and be home safe.

Finally, only then, could I return to bed, relax, and go to sleep for whatever hours were left until morning.

INSOMNIA DUE TO PAIN

The roots of my insomnia run deep. Those boyhood nights with my dad started a lifetime of anxiety-related sleeplessness. Decades later, I have never shaken the dread I feel as I try to fall sleep. Add my chronic pain and slumber is all the harder.

Chronic pain can be accompanied by several comorbidities, among them depression (see chapter 10). One less-talked-about condition is what sufferers call "painsomnia." It's not a medical term; it's just one that those of us with chronic insomnia use to capture the problem of sleeplessness when our bodies hurt.

"Like many aspects of health and wellness, the relationship between pain and sleep is bidirectional," says Robert Roy Britt, author of *Make Sleep Your Superpower: A Guide to Greater Health, Happiness & Productivity* (and, as full disclosure, my editor at *Wise & Well*). "If you're in pain, good sleep can be hard to come by, and poor sleep exacerbates pain. The reverse is true too: If you can find ways to sleep better, you can alleviate pain, and alleviating pain can improve sleep duration and quality."

How widespread is this problem? A 2012 study put the rate of insomnia among people with chronic lower back pain at an astounding 78%, meaning that about four out of five chronic pain sufferers may have trouble sleeping.

Another study published in the journal *Pain Medicine* and recently reported by clinicalpainadvisor.com, showed relative consistency in rates of insomnia among chronic pain sufferers. In a meta-analysis of 19,000 pain patients the researchers found about 60% of Asian people in the study had pain-related insomnia. The rate for Black and for white people was around 50%. Data for Hispanic, Native American, and Pacific Islander people were not reported.

MY SLEEPLESS LIFE

Most nights, I toss and turn despite taking sleeping pills. As I attempt to sleep, the pain gnaws at me. Unable to relax, I begin to wander from thought to thought about how my life and the world are going. This is generally accompanied by a gurgling gut reflecting the anxiety, echoed from childhood, I feel as I lie there.

I turn on my right side, then, after several minutes, on my left, wracked by stubborn consciousness. On good nights, I achieve something of a deep doze that gets me to morning. Weirdly, as dawn breaks, I often have cinematic dreams about my family or my former worklife.

I almost never feel rested during the day; indeed, most mornings I doze in my La-Z-Boy before the caffeine infusion of a couple of Diet Cokes kicks in.

When I do sleep, I snore like a boar. I likely have sleep apnea. I did a sleep test once, staying overnight in a lab with electrodes hooked up to me, and hated the experience, making me reluctant to try again. I used a CPAP machine for a long time but didn't see much result. I stopped because of the bulky hose and mask. I haven't returned to a sleep doctor because the hassle outweighs my misery.

I admit I have lousy sleep hygiene. I usually stay up well into late night television, a bit because of the terror of failing to sleep no matter how tired I get. I stay on devices too late: Reels is too addictive. I use a sleep mask to keep the room dark, but it ends up floating all over the bed as I flop and flip.

"I snore like a boar."

(What's the old joke? "I'll do anything to lose weight except eat right and exercise.")

Further, I "write" in my sleep, that is, my mind becomes fixated on what I'm working on during the day and thoughts about phrases float into my head. I sometimes take notes on my phone to capture brilliant points, but in the morning they mostly turn out to be nonsense. Or I'll get focused on a weird problem; last night it was how to coat my bones with silicon to protect them from disease.

(Huh? That doesn't make sense now but it did in the haze of night. Told you it is weird).

SLEEP IS FUNDAMENTAL

Because of my poor habits, I often miss out on one of the essentials of life, one that likely affects every other aspect of my health.

"Good sleep is one of the pillars of wellness, along with physical activity, healthy eating, and strong relationships," Britt says. "Sleep is foundational to all aspects of physical and mental health and longevity. As with air, water and food, we simply cannot function without sleep. And when sleep is good, all aspects of life get better."

When we sleep well, he adds, "we can be more creative, more productive. We'll get things done, which leaves more time and energy to do the fun things in life." That makes for good days, which keeps stress and anxiety at bay. "Better days lead to better nights, and better nights fuel better days. It's a powerful cycle."

An article in *The Atlantic* titled "Why Can't Americans Sleep?" called insomnia a public-health emergency. Author Jennifer Senior detailed its terrors:

"Three things are crucial for improving sleep."

I've already got a multivolume fright compendium in my head of all the terrible things that can happen when sleep eludes you or you elude it. You will die of a heart attack or a stroke. You will become cognitively compromised and possibly dement. Your weight will climb, your mood will collapse, the ramparts of your immune system will crumble. If you rely on medication for relief, you're doing your disorder all wrong — you're getting the wrong kind of sleep, an unnatural sleep, and addiction surely awaits; heaven help you and that horse of Xanax you rode in on.

WHAT TO DO ABOUT PAINSOMNIA

Three things are crucial for improving sleep if you have pain, according to Britt.

First, do everything you can to alleviate the pain. "I know that for many people, chronic pain is intractable, and you've tried everything," Britt says. "But for others, it can be a problem that's being ignored rather than properly treated. Get the pain resolved, and sleep will likely take care of itself."

Above all, Britt advises, seek pain treatments involving physical activity. "Many modern ailments (including some types of chronic pain) can be traced back to inactivity. If you are able to exercise — any sort of activity — it's well worth giving it a try, with advice from a physician of course, before turning to medications."

If you're on any prescription drugs, find out if sleep problems are a known side effect, and if so, discuss that with your physician. If insomnia persists, see a sleep specialist and do a sleep study (it's really not that bad).

Second, if nothing resolves your chronic pain, work on sleep hygiene, which refers to the process of readying for bed: "Set and stick to a consistent bedtime, spend as much time outside as you can, especially early in the morning (natural daylight keeps your body clock well-timed), be physically active, eat a healthy diet, avoid alcohol, avoid caffeine after mid-day, and give yourself a good hour or so of low-stress wind-down time before bed," says Britt.

Third, work on your mental health so that anxiety and stress from pain are minimized. "When we're in pain, we worry that it'll never end," says Britt. "Such rumination is kryptonite defeating powerful sleep."

Many are helped by mindfulness meditation, he adds.

"I used to sleep like a baby," Britt reports. "But in my 50s, I developed pain-related trouble sleeping." He would get pain in his hips and lower back that caused him to wake several times a night, stiff and sore and needing to roll over. The pain made it hard to go back to sleep. He tried multiple mattresses, and finally found a body pillow that helped.

"But I still could sleep comfortably only on one side. Then I discovered yoga. By strengthening my whole body — particularly the core — my pain was reduced to a minimum, and I sleep like a baby again. The lesson I learned, which contributed to my motivation to write my book: Never give up on good sleep."

I've taken Britt's advice to heart and I'm determined not to give up on slumber. But I also have a backup plan.

If all else fails, I'll become a vampire.

Pain Points

"The concept of 'painsomnia' really resonates, particularly the bidirectional link you and the expert describe. A bad night of sleep definitely seems to turn up the volume on any physical discomfort the next day. It's the mental part that feels so hard to untangle. The anxiety and the rumination you mentioned often feel like their own separate issue that just uses the pain as fuel." —Dr. Savio Pereira

Pain Points are comments on this essay as it appeared originally on Medium.com. They are solely the opinions of the commentators and do not necessarily reflect the views of the book author or publisher.

9

Pain Dysmorphia

My sense of self is altered, and I'm coming to grips with who I really am

When I sit with a friend having brunch at our local First Watch, I am mostly comfortable.

I look, chat, and feel "normal," like the others in the restaurant. I talk about our church, my friend's work, how my writing is going. Inside my head, I am interesting and, perhaps, at times, even charming. My friend and I wrap up the conversation and make plans to get together again.

Then it happens. I struggle to push myself up from the seat and steady myself with my cane. I tell my friend to go ahead first because I don't want her to see me doing my own version of "walking." It can be described only as hobbling along, as I hunch over and take tentative steps forward.

> *"I fear that [they] judge me as broken."*

I don't really know how she thinks of me when I walk, but I fear that she and the others in the place judge me as broken. Or, worse, they may pity me.

My sense of self as a strong, intelligent person is warped by my pain.

This disconnect between how I view myself in my mind and how I present to the world is just one aspect of what I've coined "pain dysmorphia."

WHAT IS DYSMORPHIA?

The reason I hobble when I walk is my genetic disease that deformed my joints and bones. My enduring hurt affects my body inside and out; I wrestle with the dysmorphia it brings.

Traditionally, the word "dysmorphia" has referred to self-image that is

Becoming More Me

How can I resolve my pain dysmorphia?

I'm trying to reconcile my inner and outer selves by creating then following a handful of strategies to address it.

If you are similarly afflicted — whether due to chronic pain or some other condition — I offer these ideas:

Don't fight it
In popular culture, looking abnormal is something you battle. Don't agree? For evidence, see the untold number of products aimed at making you look socially presentable, from fashion to Botox. I am giving up fighting my pain and am working to just accept it.

Be present
My pain dysmorphia is worst when I sit still and obsess about who I am. It's less prevalent when I'm present with whatever I'm doing, such as writing this book or having lunch with a friend. It's not repressing the dysmorphia; it's living the life I (and you) have today to the fullest.

Think about what you can do, rather than what you can't
In my head, I have a lifetime of fascinating experiences and harmful trauma to process. I try not to cling to the past and attempt to replay it. I

incongruent with what people see in the mirror, thus causing difficulties coping with life and sometimes physical damage and illnesses.

Further, explains Thomas Rutledge, PhD, in an article for *Psychology Today*:

In the field of mental health, perhaps the most famous example of the difficulty seeing ourselves objectively is a condition called body dysmorphia. Body dysmorphia is diagnosed when a person perceives flaws in their body or appearance to a degree that causes dysfunction or even physical harm. This condition can take many forms: underweight people can perceive themselves as fat; healthy or even well-muscled people can perceive themselves as small or weak; and people of average or even above-average attractiveness can perceive themselves as disgusting or ugly. Importantly, people with body dysmorphia are usually impervious to objective evidence and suffer the profound emotional and physical repercussions of their distorted self-perceptions.

Body dysmorphia, however, is just one narrow manifestation of our ability to create dysfunctional self-illusions. Characterizing dysmorphia more broadly as an enduring state of negative emotions and behaviors resulting from misperceptions about the self, for example, dysmorphia possesses faces and forms so numerous as to affect people in every category of age, race, gender, and social strata of our society.

So, dysmorphia can apply to anyone who experiences the difference between inner and outer self. That includes me and, perhaps, many of the other 60 million American adults who live in chronic pain.

STRUGGLING WITH PAIN DYSMORPHIA

The internet doesn't recognize the concept of pain

dysmorphia. A search for that phrase turns up no references.

I don't have a classic case of body dysmorphia, but I believe I have another version related to the damage pain has done to me, mentally and physically.

I define pain dysmorphia as the clash between what I would like to be, a hale and healthy person, and what I actually am, hurt and disabled.

I bet other chronic pain sufferers can relate, as though their bodies have betrayed them. Many of us, including those whose pain is invisible, feel a disconnect between our self-image and how we really feel.

My version of pain dysmorphia isn't that I can't see reality; I just contend with what's happened to me compared to my inner sense of self. My genetic disease and the pain that goes with it have left me mostly sedentary, feeling trapped. When I do get around, I use a cane or a wheelchair. My gait is abnormal, more of a jerking motion than ambling. Each step brings pain, which likely shows in my body language and face.

Some of this comes with age, of course, but I've struggled with dysmorphia because of my pain for decades.

I can't quite resolve who I really am with the person I see myself as.

This does not compute.

THE PAIN DYSMORPHIA GAP

My pain dysmorphia isn't about eternal youth. I appreciate aging. But there is a gap between how I see myself in my mind and what I see in the mirror each day. It's akin to well-recognized psychological phenomenon called "subjective age," whereby many

concentrate on what I can do now rather than the things I've had to set aside as I've aged, like making a hook shot or swimming in the ocean.

Build an identity outside your pain
For me, pain is a constant, but I don't let it become my whole identity. I am not just a disabled pain sufferer, but a husband, father, grandfather, writer, TV and movie watcher, and fan of just about anything that can be called a spectator sport. I have more to offer the world than being a pain sufferer.

Hang out with others in pain
I've gotten lots of help in dealing with my pain from online peer support groups offered by the U.S. Pain Foundation or Chronic Pain Anonymous (see Sources of Solace). I get to see others who suffer and may also be confronting the difference between their inner and outer selves.

This helps normalize how I see other people in pain. In these groups, I don't ever have to stress because I'm not trying to present an unrealistic version of myself.

people feel, in their hearts and minds, about 20% younger than what the mirror says.

In my mind, I'm eternally 30-something — youngish, strong, and smart. I move easily, playing racquetball with my boss and mentor, touring European capitals, and completing complex home improvement projects.

Inside, I am cool like I was decades ago; in reality, I am past my "use by" date. (This just in: My wife reports I was *never* cool.) My inner self is bursting with energy to help the world, but practically speaking I want to lie down to stop the pain.

For me, pain dysmorphia causes cognitive dissonance between the person I see in my mind's eye and the actual me.

How do you see yourself? Is it congruent with who you actually are? Ditch the dysmorphia. Accept that person in the mirror as the real you.

Pain Points

"[Use] something to indicate who you are, right from the beginning. It's daunting at first, but it's much better than trying to mask the pain. … Maybe [put on] a pin that says, 'Invisible disability never looked so fabulous.'" —Jenn Biddle

"I've also been in pain since my teens. But mine was related to my art — dance (ballet, in particular). … I had a colleague (mentor), who, when I asked, 'Why does it have to be so painful?' He replied, 'That just means you're alive.' Lately, I've practiced loving and luxuriating in my pain (rather than resisting it). … Example: I fell down the stairs last year. … I hobbled like a broken jalopy in a cartoon for about 24 hours. One moment, I thought, *If I were one of my students, what would I say?* I'd say, 'Just tell your legs to stand you up.' So, I told my right leg and made it stand me straight up tall. Then, the — excruciating — left leg and made it stand me up tall. In four such steps, 98% of all the debilitating pain of the last 24 hours disintegrated into thin air. … We each have an inner genius who can help find whatever we look for (or expect). … I get to choose." —Ian Howard

Pain Points are comments on this essay as it appeared originally on Medium.com. They are solely the opinion of the commentators and do not necessarily reflect the views of the book author or publisher.

PAIN PROFILE

Was Her Pain Dismissed?

After suffering serious burns, my wife is coming to terms with chronic hurt

My wife knew she was in trouble, just not how much.

Just before Thanksgiving in 2020, I returned home from a pool workout to discover MeK weeping on a couch in our home in East Tennessee. She held her right arm close to her chest.

She'd just donated blood, something she'd done since she was 17 years old. At age 59, she had once again taken part in the MEDIC blood drive held annually before the Tennessee Vols vs. Kentucky Wildcats college football game.

Everything went normally until she arrived back at our empty house. She began feeling lightheaded, which she took as hunger.

"I ate a snack after donating, but MEDIC was out of my usual peanut butter crackers," she recalls. "I settled for a Little Debby oatmeal cookie. At home, I decided to make popcorn on our flat-top electric stove." (Popcorn is her drug of choice.)

As she turned on the front burner, put cooking oil in a pan, and coated its bottom with kernels, things suddenly went black.

> *"Looking closer, she realized the shirt was burned, the fabric fused into her skin."*

BURNING SENSATION

Seconds later, MeK awoke on the hard tile floor in front of the stove. She didn't hurt, though her right arm felt icy cold. She lifted it and noticed the bottom half of her shirt sleeve was torn. Looking closer, she realized the shirt was burned, the fabric fused into her skin.

Then she became aware of the burning-fabric-skin-oil odor in the kitchen. "The pain started to register," MeK says. "My right forearm went from freezing to being stabbed with a thousand hot needles."

MeK managed to crawl her way onto the couch, where she'd left her iPhone.

She texted me "Help!" but my phone was in the gym locker, and I didn't check it while driving home.

I opened the front door and then heard someone faintly calling my name. I found MeK suffering on that couch. I tried to touch her arm, but she recoiled.

"We're going to the ER now," I said.

UNDERPLAYING HER INJURY

Later, we pieced together what likely happened.

While fainting because of the loss of blood from the donation (which can happen suddenly), MeK had apparently reached out to steady herself on the stove. She must have dragged her right hand and forearm across the hot burner as she fell, fusing her polyester shirt onto her skin from elbow to palm.

After a few moments, she regained consciousness, but following her Irish Catholic born-not-to-bother-anyone upbringing, she chose not to call 911. MeK says:

> *I naturally underplay any injury or illness. Growing up, my parents, brothers, and I lived with my aunt, who was the operating room head nurse at our local hospital. Unless something was broken or bleeding uncontrollably, she thought any childhood injuries weren't worthy of a doctor or hospital visit. But, since this pain was hitting full force, I agreed to go to the ER.*

After we waited awhile, the doctor at our local hospital emergency department dismissed MeK's burns, sending us home with ointment for the wound.

A week later, the blistered tissue hadn't healed, in fact looked much worse, and MeK was in searing pain. Fortunately, our youngest daughter shared a photo of the injury with a friend whose stepfather is a military surgeon.

He was shocked. He told MeK that the burn looked infected and that she should immediately get to the trauma center at the University of Tennessee Medical Center in Knoxville.

When doctors there looked at the wound, they too were alarmed. They decided her situation was beyond even the trauma center's capabilities and told MeK she needed to go to the burn unit at Vanderbilt University in Nashville, three hours away, as soon as possible.

"The docs at UT and Vanderbilt agreed that the tissue on my forearm was infected and dying off," MeK says. "They said I could have lost my arm."

DOCTORS DEBRIDE THE BURN

At Vanderbilt University Medical Center, doctors diagnosed MeK with third-degree burns. She at once underwent emergency surgery to graft skin from a cadaver donor onto her arm. The surgeon "debrided" the wound, meaning he scraped and gouged out the dying skin and infected tissue.

> *"[The doctors] said I could have lost my arm."*

A couple of days later, after MeK received antibiotics, a surgeon did a second graft. He harvested a section of skin from her front right thigh and replanted it onto her right hand and forearm. The recovery was painful, involving not just caring for the original burns but also for the new 4- by 8-inch raging-red wound on her leg.

Though grateful for the care, throughout the whole experience MeK found that doctors and other healthcare workers seemed to underplay her condition and pain as not that bad — an attitude that she, as a woman, had experienced before:

> *Throughout my life, it's usually the male physicians who have disregarded or explained away my symptoms such as debilitating headaches, periodic blood pressure spikes, fatigue, and dizziness as 'stress' or, more precisely, 'the stress of taking care of kids and a husband.'*

Instead of ordering diagnostic tests, doctors would instruct her to "go for a walk," "get more rest," or another version of the unstated message, "You're the one causing your symptoms, so you're the only one who can make them go away."

This happens to women a lot. They are often dissed, dismissed, and gaslit about their pain (see chapter 19).

THE GENDER PAIN GAP

Such was the conclusion of a 2024 study of 2,040 women and men in Australia by Nurofen:

> *There is a Gender Pain Gap affecting the lives of women across Australia, with*

55% of women feeling they have had their pain ignored or dismissed compared with 48% of men. Moreover, among those who felt that way, 32% of women versus 20% of men believe it was because their general practitioner didn't take their pain seriously.

It goes on to say that, among respondents who believe the gender pain gap exists, about half think that's because women are seen as more emotional than men. About the same amount say females are expected to naturally feel more pain. Other reasons include the ideas that they have hormones different from males, women and men have dissimilar pain tolerance, and women's pain tends to be downplayed as psychological, as MeK's often was.

"People see women as being hysterical but see men as stoic, so for a man to be in pain it must be really bad," says Bill Laughey, MD, Nurofen's in-house general practitioner and the senior medical scientist at its parent company, Reckitt, in a *Marie Claire Australia* article. "People make corrections in their heads when they hear a pain story. For women, [they] bring it down a bit: 'Oh, you're saying a 7 out of 10? It's probably a 5.' And for a man, there's the temptation to add one on. It's such an unfair contradistinction. It's a bias, it's not a fact."

MEK FINALLY FINDS RELIEF

About four months after MeK's accident, she and I moved from Tennessee to suburban Philadelphia, in part so she could be a caregiver for our first granddaughter. Her hand and forearm still seared with constant pain, the burn tight from scarring.

Searching for relief, she phoned for an appointment with a reconstructive surgeon pioneering a new type of CO_2 laser surgery at the now closed Crozer-Chester Medical Center burn center in Chester, Pennsylvania. The procedure essentially pokes minute holes in the scars to loosen them and increase mobility. MeK says:

For the first time in the whole burn nightmare, I finally felt heard, seen, and taken seriously. All it took was one look at my scarred, frozen hand, wrist, and forearm, and the surgeon and his team said they could help. Moreover, they were angry and saddened that I hadn't received the right aftercare in Tennessee. Thanks to the resulting laser procedures, I've regained significant function in my fingers, wrist, and hand. My pain level has gone down substantially.

Years after the accident, MeK still resists thinking of herself as someone who experiences chronic pain, due in part to her "rub-dirt-on-it" upbringing.

"Annoying," "stiff," and "tight" are typically the adjectives she uses to describe how her skin feels now that the burns, skin graft, and laser treatments have healed. But, by the afternoon each day, her skin tightness morphs into pain — dull and constant at times, stabbing on occasion.

For this reason, I reassure her that she has indeed joined me as one of the more than 60 million American adults who live in chronic pain.

ASSESSING HER EXPERIENCE

Looking back, from my initial trip to the emergency room through my first physical and occupational therapy visits after getting the grafts. I got this sense from most of the healthcare providers that my burns weren't all that terrible. As a woman, I believed them — even though the pain and limited hand, wrist, and forearm function I experienced told a different story. I've been conditioned by the healthcare system not to listen to my body, because, obviously, since I'm a woman, my body and my brain can't be trusted.

Like many women, MeK learned early to downplay her pain. Her inclination to minimize her own discomfort and soldier on, she believes, is a direct result of watching how her mother responded to pain, sickness, and injury.

She vividly remembers a time seeing her mom pouring a pot of scalding hot water into a colander in the sink to drain spaghetti and having a wave of that water splash up on her. Her mother jumped back slightly and made a grunting sound but never stopped draining the water from the pot. It was only after she put the drained spaghetti into a bowl that she lifted her shirt to calmly examine her skin. Where the water had splashed was bright red and obviously painful (and eventually blistered), but she never complained.

> "Obviously, since I'm a woman, my body and my brain can't be trusted."

"I recall the way she silently endured her injury with the task at hand," MeK says.

And that is what MeK does anytime she accidentally slices her finger while chopping veggies, bops her head on a doorway while carrying our squirmy granddaughter, or experiences any of the other common daily injuries that befall women — or, yes, some men — as they cook and clean, walk dogs, and take care of their homes and families.

"Pain and sickness are part of the territory when you're a mom or a grandma.

You just deal with it," she says.

MeK resisted for a while but finally has accepted that chronic pain will be part of her life. Her experience has inspired her to be more activist about her healthcare.

She concludes: "I'm beginning to trust my instincts and speak up for myself."

10

My Skin's Too Tight

*Living with the double burdens of
chronic pain and depression*

I hit rock bottom when I wept watching *Xena: Warrior Princess*.

It was June 18, 2001. (I know because I just looked it up on IMDb.) I'd been a fan of the television series for years (the show premiered in 1995), in no small part because of lead Kiwi actress Lucy Lawless clad in leather. Now it was coming to an end.

In the series finale, Xena is dead, and despite heroic but fruitless efforts to resurrect her, the warrior princess's implied lover, Gabrielle, is left alone. The scene that got to me is the final one, with a long shot from the sky showing the latter standing solo on the bow of a ship sailing into some new unknown life. Alone. All alone.

My reaction was disproportionate to the cheesy made-for-syndicated-TV moment. But I could feel the heartbreak, loneliness, and loss. I cried at the thought of the two lovers separated — one dead and the other left to live on without her.

> *"[The doctor] diagnosed me with major depression."*

I knew it was silly to weep at a fantasy TV show, but something deeper was going on inside me. Even though I was surrounded by people — my wife, my three daughters, my mother and brother, my friends, my coworkers — I felt so alone.

A few months later, after 9/11 and the additional sadness it brought, I finally went to a psychiatrist. He diagnosed me with major depression. The clinical kind. The one that goes beyond having the blues.

I also had, and still do, chronic pain syndrome, thanks to the MED that caused

Decreasing Depression

Depression is often overlooked in chronic pain treatment, though over time more physicians are taking a holistic "biopsychosocial" approach to pain (see chapter 26). I responded well to medicine for depression, but I still have it and go through periodic episodes of sadness and ennui. I also practice other ways to beat the blues, including these:

Therapy
I see a psychologist with whom I talk about my pain. I mostly come away from these discussions more optimistic. Other sufferers may be similarly helped. For instance, research reported in *Pain Medicine News* that interventions that reduce catastrophizing, something that many chronic pain sufferers are prone to, can help cut pain scores.

Get outside
Nature is healing. Even if you need to experience it using a wheelchair, find an accessible national or state park and have someone push you, the way my wife pushes me (see chapter 2). It's more difficult to be depressed when you take in the wonder around you.

Sleep
"Painsomnia" (see chapter 16) is real and it may be tough to get enough sleep when you are in chronic pain. Still, high-quality rest can reduce depression symptoms.

my joints to deform, resulting in a constant grind when I move my body. It wears me down.

HAND IN HAND

Chronic pain and depression go hand in hand. According to a literature study published by the *Journal of the American Medical Association* (*JAMA Internal Medicine*), patients in pain are more likely to be depressed than patients not in pain. At the same time, depressed people report more pain than people not depressed.

In addition, the study reported that individuals with long-term chronic pain are three times more likely to be depressed than those without pain. The paper compared rates of depression in various settings and found, for example, that an average of 56% of patients at orthopedic or rheumatology clinics were depressed.

WHAT IS DEPRESSION LIKE?

How do I describe what it is to be clinically depressed?

Let's go to an expert first. According to the Mayo Clinic website:

> *Depression ranges in seriousness from mild, temporary episodes of sadness to severe, persistent depression. Clinical depression is the more severe form of depression, also known as major depression or major depressive disorder. It isn't the same as depression caused by a loss, such as the death of a loved one, or a medical condition, such as a thyroid disorder.*

That definition doesn't capture the reality of depression as I felt it.

(A note: The following deals with suicide. If you feel suicidal or are thinking about self-harm, please stop reading and immediately call or text the 988 Suicide and Crisis Lifeline at 988. Don't wait. Talk to someone.)

In November 1992, I happened to read an article in *The New York Times Magazine*. Headlined "Most Likely to Succeed," it was about Frank Aller, a longtime friend of Bill Clinton's, predating his presidency. Aller and Clinton were Rhodes scholars together at Oxford University in England in the '60s. A few years later, in 1971, Aller shot himself in the head with a .22 caliber pistol in his hometown of Spokane, Washington.

The article linked his suicide to his decision to avoid the Vietnam draft and talked about how it bedeviled him. But that angle didn't capture the deeper reality of Aller's life as a brilliant super-achiever who "took it all too seriously," according to a friend. Though some in his circle speculated that he couldn't live with being called a draft dodger, the women in his life gave a subtler picture that led me to think he had clinical depression.

In the article, there was a quote from Aller's friend Jan Brenning, who confessed she couldn't figure out why Aller took his life, but observed, "He was caught in skin that had gotten too tight."

The idea of "skin too tight" has stayed with me through the decades since then. To me, it sums up what I felt at the worst of my depression, a terrible sense of being suffocated in my own body.

PHYSICAL AND PSYCHOLOGICAL

I am not a doctor or medical professional and am simply speaking from my own experience, but I believe I am dealing primarily with physical depression, some malfunction in the brain that causes feelings of hopelessness. Something about my body chemistry is off-kilter, perhaps due to my MED,

Listen to music
Chappell Roan or Taylor Swift may be able to relieve chronic pain and depression. A 2025 study showed that music therapy effectively reduces these conditions.

Exercise
Moving is easier said than done for chronic pain sufferers (believe me, I know), but, as illogical as it sounds, exercise is a good prescription for reducing pain, as research published in 2025 in the *Journal of Affective Disorders* showed.

Remember: Movement is medicine (see Pain Profile: Movement Is Medicine).

and it caused such symptoms as an all-encompassing feeling of being trapped, unable to experience much joy, with persistent thoughts that all is not right with the world. I also have some degree of psychological depression.

Depression can be dealt with through medication, therapy, exercise, acupuncture, and other methods. I was lucky. After some trial and, mostly, error, my psychiatrist got me on an effective antidepressant. (Antidepressants are also sometimes given to chronic pain patients.)

He warned me that these drugs work slowly, so I mustn't be an impatient patient. That wasn't the case for me. From the first day I took this new drug I felt better.

> *"The idea of 'skin too tight' has stayed with me."*

It wasn't euphoria. Rather, it was an absence of the crushing feeling that I'd experienced for so long. I also got relief by talking with counselors and by exercising as much as my chronic pain allows.

(Remember: I am not a doctor and am not advising you to take any drug or supplement to deal with pain or depression. Always consult a physician about any treatment you are considering.)

WHAT SCIENCE SAYS

Study after study confirms the link between chronic pain and depression. For example, a meta-analysis of 375 studies on chronic pain and mood, reported in the JAMA Open Network, puts the rate of chronic pain sufferers who also have clinically significant depression and anxiety at 40%.

That means there are about two in five chronic pain sufferers who are also depressed. The research showed people with fibromyalgia are most likely to be depressed, at 54%. The least likely are those with arthritis, at about 30%. Women and young people with pain are particularly prone to depression.

Other fascinating research, published in *Science Advances* and released in 2025, showed that the more places in the body sufferers hurt, the greater their chances of depression. It also found that depression may be linked to chronic inflammation.

Another study by the University College London investigated the timing of pain and depression. It revealed that middle-aged and senior adults who have pain "are more likely to have had worsening symptoms of depression up to eight years before the pain began." In other words, depression earlier in life may predict chronic pain later.

UNDER CONTROL

Now, two decades later, my clinical depression is mostly under control thanks to medication, but often my intractable chronic pain can make me feel hopeless, weary, and threatened.

When this happens, I think about my greatest strength: resilience. I'm terrific at the ability to endure what life throws at me, a trait I share with many chronic pain and depression sufferers. In my experience, it takes courage, grit, and the help of medical professionals, friends, and family to not let sadness overtake you when you have enduring physical and emotional hurt.

In 2024, in a Zoom pain support group, the moderator asked everyone to write what we would tell others with the same disease. I thought about my twin burdens of pain and depression. I wrote:

It sucks but it doesn't have to destroy your life. There are ways of coping and thriving. Rely on your resilience. Get information. Be an advocate for yourself with family, doctors, and others.

You are not your illness. It doesn't define you.

Pain Points

"Resilience. That's the win." —Michele Cambardella

Pain Points are comments on this essay as it appeared originally on Medium.com. They are solely the opinion of the commentators and do not necessarily reflect the views of the book author or publisher.

11

Post-Op Proposal

How I got engaged after my first hip replacement — at age 27

The nurse looked shocked as she entered the room.

She checked the chart again, then raised her eyes to stare skeptically at me lying in a bed at St. Mary's Hospital in Knoxville, Tennessee, in August 1985.

"I thought there was a typo with your age, honey," she finally said. "I figured you'd be 72."

"Nope," I replied. "It's right. I'm 27."

"But you're here for a hip replacement," the nurse added. "We usually don't do them in someone your age."

My then girlfriend, now my wife, MeK, smiled at the exchange as she stood at my bedside.

Apologetically, I said to the nurse, "Sorry," somehow ashamed that I was too young for the operation I was to have the next day.

> *"My hip had hurt for years as it degenerated due to my genetic disease."*

My hip had hurt for years as it degenerated due to my genetic disease. Bone ground on bone, causing intense pain. It was like mismatched gears rubbing against each other, slowly grating the teeth to nubs. This happened throughout my body — to my ankles, knees, shoulders, and so on — but it evolved worst in the weight-bearing hips.

I was always an active kid, playing Little League (badly) and pick-up basketball (slightly better), weight-lifting in PE class, and swimming in a neighbor kid's pool, but I was doing damage to my joints.

"By my 20s, I had put a lot of mileage on my body."

In fourth grade at Enadia Way Elementary School in Canoga Park, California, I wore a full foot-to-hip brace on my left leg designed to prevent the hip joint from dislocating. As the other kids ran around during recess, I sat on a shaded bench listening to Paul Revere and the Raiders on a Craig tape player my teacher let me bring to school.

This turned out to be a wasted year. The brace didn't help my condition much and before long, I'd done away with it and returned to furiously wrestling in the pool and boisterously enjoying made-up games with my brother and friends.

EXISTENTIAL DREAD

By my 20s, I had put a lot of mileage on my body and now I needed both hips replaced, starting with the left side.

My orthopedic surgeon, the late Frank Gray, had the cockiness of a fighter pilot. He promised me that the replacements would erase my pain, giving me a new life — at least for 15 to 20 years. Then I'd need the hips revised as the prostheses wore out.

Staying in the hospital the night before surgery, I was nervous — bad things can always happen when you go under anesthesia — but the pain I had endured was so terrible that I had no choice. Over the previous months, I consulted with MeK and we decided to go for it.

I had moved to Knoxville in 1980 for a job as a writer-editor after I graduated from Boston University. MeK and I first got together in 1982, when she was a "return" (an intern who'd come back for a second summer) at my employer, 13–30 Corp, which specialized in publications for teens and young adults. We dated long distance until she got a full-time job there a couple of years later.

Without her Irish Catholic parents knowing, we moved in together a few months after her arrival to a loft-bedroom apartment in the Woodgate complex on North Knoxville's Cedar Lane. It was a big decision. It reflected our commitment to each other, but we hadn't yet discussed marriage. I was young and single and more interested in drinking $1.50 Long Island Teas at local happy hours.

Now, as I struggled with existential dread about the operation and what it would take to walk again, MeK was there with me, ready to care for me as I recovered. Although some do, no one should go through such a serious surgery as a joint replacement alone. I don't recall that we had a debate about whether she would help; it just fell into place. Something in her heart must have told her that I was worth the significant work that was needed to get me back on my feet.

OOZE, GOO, AND GORE

Hip replacements are bloody affairs. (I once had an orthopedist — not Dr. Gray — confess to me that his favorite thing about his job was using power tools.)

During the operation, the surgeon uses a scalpel to cut through the flesh and muscle covering the joint. (I know this because I have a foot-long scar running from my upper thigh to my waist.)

Once he gets down to bone, he employs an electric saw to cut the head off the femur. He power-drills the screws that hold the artificial cup to the pelvis. Lower-tech hammers are used to pound the shaft of the artificial hip into the hollow core that runs down the femur's length. The addition of industrial-strength glue keeps things in place.

It's all ooze, goo, and gore. No wonder that after that hip replacement I felt like I'd been hit by a locomotive. The operation went well, but the pain was almost unbearable. I recall screaming at the nurses to "Stop!" when they rolled me onto my right side (see chapter 20). The prospect of even more hurt terrified me.

I stayed in the hospital for three days. In the 1980s, the best practice was to let patients rest and heal without activity. Today, surgeons get them up on, say, a new hip right away and sometimes send them home within hours with prescriptions for months of physical therapy to strengthen muscles and promote bone growth. Not so back then.

So, I returned home to rest. MeK and I had a bed brought to the first floor of our loft apartment. I slept downstairs while she slept upstairs. I settled in to heal with a television and remote nearby. I remember she and I watched *Live Aid* on July 13, 1985. The all-star concert (Freddie Mercury and Queen stole the show) to fight hunger in Africa was broadcast from Wembley Stadium in London and JFK Stadium in Philadelphia (where, coincidently, we moved decades later). Laid up, I watched the whole 16 hours of coverage, which ended with an amazing performance of "We Are the World."

WORLD-CLASS CAREGIVING

Throughout those days of recovery, MeK tended to me. She made meals, changed bandages, and, without complaining, emptied urinals. More than that, though, she emotionally sustained me. She encouraged me with an "It'll be okay" every time I felt a stab in the hip and fretted that something had badly gone wrong. I couldn't have recovered as well without her. Slowly I healed and was able to hobble my way around the apartment on crutches.

What she didn't know was that before the operation, I visited Markman's Jewelry at Knoxville's East Towne Mall. I picked out a $600 engagement ring, the most I could afford back then. I'd hidden it on the floor under my recovery bed. I'd take it out once in a while just to stare at it and think about how I'd ask her to marry me. I decided to do it on her upcoming birthday, August 15.

In retrospect, we'd been headed for marriage for a while, but it was when I lay in that bed recovering — just a handful of years from turning 30 — that I realized partying like I was still in college had gotten old. I thought about what I wanted in life. Her willingness to take care of me while I healed signaled how deeply she was committed to me.

> *"Spoiler alert: She said 'yes.'"*

It cemented what I already knew before the operation — that MeK was the best person I'd ever known (that's still true). Her selflessness while I was laid up didn't take any special effort. Caring came naturally to her (see chapter 24).

She wasn't a saint; I'm sure even hinting at that would have embarrassed her and come with a firm "I am not." She and I had our share of pushing the other's buttons, but I guess it's a measure of how bonded you are to someone that he or she knows exactly how to bug you.

On the evening of August 14, a Wednesday, we watched a Los Angeles Dodgers game that lasted past midnight on the East Coast. As the clock struck midnight, making it officially her birthday, I was so excited about proposing that I couldn't wait another minute.

I clicked off the TV. (MeK knew something serious was up, as I'd never turn off a game until the last out was recorded.) I leaned over to grab the ring from the floor, then moved to the end of the bed where she sat. Without ceremony, I blurted out, "Will you marry me?"

MORE SURGERIES

Spoiler alert: She said "yes" immediately. I had gotten other presents for her birthday too, including a plane ticket for her to visit her parents, who lived in the house she grew up in, in the Boston area. On Friday, she flew home and had the whole wedding, which we would hold in Rockport and Gloucester, Massachusetts, planned by the time she returned from the weekend.

This is the story of my first joint replacement. I say "first" because I've had eight in all. Months after the left hip, I had my right done.

Around the turn of the millennium, both hip replacements had worn out and I needed "revisions." Then, in the 2010s, my feet had become so deformed that I walked on the outside edges, causing them to bend at a 45-degree angle to the ankle. I had both ankles fused to return my feet to being flat on the floor. Within the next few years, I also had both knees and both shoulders replaced.

MeK was there through it all, caring for me again and again. She and I will be married 40 years in 2026, assuming she doesn't surprise me with a divorce.

I now walk with a cane for short distances and use a wheelchair for longer ones. MeK pushes me around when we visit places like state parks with accessible walking paths. (See chapter 24). We've had our ups and downs through surgeries and a lifetime of career and family milestones — including my forced retirement due to disability at age 53 (see chapter 4) — but we've never quit on each other.

Recently, I told her she's still the best person I know.

She replied: "You need to get out more."

12

The Disability Paradox

*If you think people with handicaps
lead terrible lives, think again*

Regardless of what you've read in this book, I am not miserable.

Sure, as I've written, I live with chronic pain. So do about 60 million American adults, more than 21 million of whom have high impact chronic pain, like me.

My rare genetic disease causes osteoarthritis throughout the body. It crashed my career as a writer, editor, and marketer (see chapter 4). I estimate my condition cost me $2 million (see chapter 5).

In this book, I explore what it's really like to live in chronic pain, including the physical and psychological effects. But I worry that I've given the false impression that my life, and those of other chronic pain sufferers, is nothing but a pitiful existence.

"Able-bodied people think the disabled lead terrible lives."

It's not. Nor is that true of a majority of people with disabilities, says a seminal study included in the National Library of Medicine.

Unfortunately, physicians and the public don't understand that happiness and handicaps can coexist. This is called "the disability paradox," so coined by researchers around the turn of the millennium.

ESSENCE OF THE PARADOX

The essence of the paradox: Able-bodied people think the disabled lead terrible lives. Those of us who are handicapped disagree and report that, while our lives are sometimes sad, they are generally satisfying and can be joyous, like everyone else's.

Nearly 30% of American adults have some kind of disability. Our burdens may be mental or physical; some are slight and some are fatal. Our conditions are hereditary or acquired. Our lives can be a constant struggle.

"Humans tend to be resilient." We are often invisible, except if we have physical differences. We live within limits on what we can do; for me, even taking a shower is a bit of a trial. We are as ambitious as the able-bodied, but we understand some doors are closed to us. (I've given up trying to manifest an NBA career.)

We are embarrassed to ask for help, but consideration is forever appreciated. A door held open is always welcome.

We may, like me, use canes and wheelchairs, making us stand out in public. We hate stairs and stares.

RESILIENCE IS HUMAN

But humans tend to be resilient. We wouldn't have survived as a species if we weren't. Whether by nature or nurture, we tend to bounce back from difficulties and get on with our lives.

"We neglect to consider the power of our psychological immune systems, coping strategies, and resilience," says Kathleen Bogart, PhD, professor of psychology, Oregon State University, in an essay in *Psychology Today*.

When it comes to coping, people with disabilities are no different from others. We work, have relationships, and celebrate, just like the able-bodied. We do mundane things like shop for groceries, get haircuts, work out at the gym, drive, and fight with our partners.

We find ways to manage our conditions. We learn. We react. We adapt. In short, we live our lives, like everyone else.

That's the story of humanity, even for those who face barriers.

LIVING DISABLED, LIVING WELL

Though we suffer, we don't want your pity or a "Bless your heart."

We want you to see us as full people, maybe with heavier crosses to bear than most, but with potential, passion, and pride. Overall, our lives are valuable, despite what people think.

Allen Rucker is a man who lives with paralysis. He explains the disability paradox in an essay on the Christopher and Dana Reeve Foundation website:

> *Multiple peer-reviewed studies have shown, and legions of disabled people confirm, that many of us thought of as damaged goods experience a satisfying or excellent quality of life, that we find purpose, joy, love, and self-worth in equal or even greater measure than many others. We live with limitations and even periodic pain and suffering and yet forge ahead to make life work in wondrous ways even though we are perceived to be permanently damaged and condemned to a bleak, forlorn fate. This is the disability paradox. You are disabled, but life is good.*

Good and bad coexisting. What a concept.

OUR BIGGEST PROBLEM

The biggest bane of disability is other people's attitudes.

Those without disabilities may reject us, stigmatize us, or ignore us because they assume our lives are not worth living.

The worst of all is when they blame us for our conditions, as though we chose to be disabled and it is some failure of moral character.

My oldest daughter, who shares my disability, had other students in high school tell her that she could just "pray away" her problem.

Explains Bogart:

> *People fear becoming disabled and pity those who do. Nondisabled people assume that people with disabilities have a worse quality of life, but this idea contradicts what many people with disabilities actually think. When asked to rate disabled people's quality of life, nondisabled people assume it is low — lower in fact than people with the disability in question rate their own quality of life. This gap between what nondisabled people believe and what people with disabilities actually experience is known as the disability paradox.*

Negative attitudes toward the disabled have consequences. When our lives are seen as less worthy, physicians, policymakers, and the public may dismiss us.

Research reported in HealthAffairs offers an example:

> *In our survey of 714 practicing US physicians nationwide, 82.4% reported that people with significant disability have worse quality of life than nondisabled*

89

people. Only 40.7% of physicians were very confident about their ability to provide the same quality of care to patients with disability, just 56.5% strongly agreed that they welcomed patients with disability into their practices, and 18.1% strongly agreed that the healthcare system often treats these patients unfairly.

The implications of these stats: Do the disabled get worse healthcare because doctors and others see us as living lesser lives?

DISABILITY DOCUMENTARY

Northern Ireland native Chris Lynch made the 2020 BBC documentary *The Disability Paradox* (available on YouTube) because he has struggled to find happiness with his handicaps. He has osteogenesis imperfecta — a congenital disease that, among other things, causes brittle bones — and uses a wheelchair.

But, "Saying that, I've been lucky as I've lived a lot. I've DJed and been supporting DJs. I've run a number of successful businesses. I'm a camera operator and an aspiring filmmaker and I've recently gained my commercial drone license," Lynch reports.

In the documentary, UK actor, writer, and activist Samantha Renke, who has the same condition as Lynch, observes:

There is definitely this disability perception gap. So nondisabled people definitely think there's been a shift because they start to see more people like me on the telly, but actually the reality is [that] disabled people still feel discriminated against, still face prejudice on a daily basis. But now we're like, no, don't bless me, you know, don't want to change me, don't think I can be cured by going to church. I am me and there's nothing to be ashamed of.

Renke is short of stature and in a wheelchair, but asserts strongly:

[My life is] pretty darn good. ... I am actually living my dream. I did exactly what I set out to do and I don't think many people can necessarily say that. ... They see me on telly, smashing it at life, like doing really well, like makes good money ... doing really well in her career ... does red carpets, has celebrity friends, yet the same people that see me still will pat me on the head and go, 'Bless you.'

"If you look at someone in a wheelchair, you think that person in a wheelchair is paying attention to being in the wheelchair," comments Paul Dolan, professor of behavioral science, London School of Economics, in the documentary. "And, of course, if they were all of the time, they would be as miserable as we would imagine them to be, [but they aren't]."

Documentarian Chris Lynch also interviews Havi Carel, a professor of philosophy at Bristol University. Carel talks about Harriet Johnson, who is a disability activist in the US, has congenital spine deformation, and uses a wheelchair:

> *[Johnson] says that she would be waiting for the light to change on the street corner and people would come up to her and say, 'If I had to live like you, I'd kill myself'.' So, the disability paradox refers to this strange sort of human psychological phenomenon where you expect people who suffer from significant illness or disability to have a much lower level of well-being than healthy or able-bodied counterparts [but] that doesn't come true in real life.*

Carel adds:

> *We view [illness] from the outside as this monolithically evil, terrible disaster, but actually, within that, there's so much nuance. And once the dust settles after the diagnosis, most people forge a way forward with whatever other things and tools — and tools of resilience — they have in their own lives.*

Documentary interviewees Stafford and Jean Lynn are married. Both use wheelchairs. Stafford was hurt in a motorcycle mishap at age 29. Jean became disabled with a spinal injury riding horseback at 17. They have a child together.

> *"I don't mean to sugarcoat disability."*

Says Jean:

> *[The accident] happened and I moved on. You [have] to move on. … I actually couldn't be happier. If I had a genie in a lamp and someone offered me to not have a disability, I don't think I would pick that. This is my life, this is my path, and it's awesome.*

I AM NOT MY DISEASE

I don't mean to sugarcoat disability. It is not something to be wished for. It is hard and often painful. But as people like Samantha Renke and Jean Lynn testify, life is good despite their handicaps.

My own experience is that my disability doesn't define me. It may be the first thing other people see. They may look at me with pity or disdain. They may try to put me in a category of "that poor man."

But I am so much more than a pathology.

My life is full of pain — but also mundane tasks, moments of joy, and fun with family.

I hurt; I love life.

I am a paradox.

Pain Points

"I've had a fear of heights since my early twenties, but do I think of how I have missed out on bungee-jumping or parachuting? We hold paradox on many things."
—Sharon Johnson

"Invisible disabilities are very challenging though. I have to break expectations all the time because I look 'normal' (whatever that means) and when I tell people I'm disabled, they blow me off or say 'Noooo, you can't be.' Then they begin to observe and experience my extreme sensitivities; they say, 'Mind over body, baby' and expect me to deal with the pain of cars and trucks and toxic cleaning products like it's nothing."
—Christina Ballew

Pain Points are comments on this essay as it appeared originally on Medium.com. They are solely the opinion of the commentators and do not necessarily reflect the views of the book author or publisher.

Part II: Understanding Chronic Pain

"You never know how strong you are until being strong is your only choice."

— Bob Marley

"Pain nourishes courage. You can't be brave if you've only had wonderful things happen to you."

— Mary Tyler Moore

"If you feel pain, you're alive. If you feel other people's pain, you're a human being."

— Leo Tolstoy

Source: **Wisdomquotes.com**

13

Defining Chronic Pain

The standard meaning misses the reality

For decades I've suffered from chronic pain.

I know how it feels inside my body, how much it affects my attitude, how it impacts every aspect of my life.

But it's hard to communicate that.

What does "chronic pain" really mean? What exactly is its definition? How can I make everyone understand what I'm talking about?

> *"The meaning of chronic pain is squishy."*

It turns out the meaning of chronic pain is squishy.

The standard definitions are like that in a book from StatPearls Publishing: "The condition encompasses a wide range of persistent discomfort lasting beyond three to six months and often originates from various sources, including injury, disease, or unknown causes."

This contrasts with "acute pain," which is the pain we feel when we hit our thumb with a hammer. Acute pain comes from physical damage, hurts for a short while, and heals.

With chronic pain, however, we are not talking about skinned knees. Phrases like "persistent discomfort" underplays what chronic pain is really like.

INADEQUATE DEFINITION
The simple definition of chronic pain based on how long it lasts is inadequate to capture the reality for sufferers. It belies the genuine desperation people with chronic pain feel.

For me, it's not simply how long but more importantly how much an individual hurts. Quantity of time is not as critical as quality of pain.

Of course, chronic pain ranges widely in severity from one person to the next. We each have our own pain threshold. Our individual pain is unique to us.

My pain is like a WWE wrestler battering my body each day.

For some people, the horrible hurt is unavoidable, untenable, and unremitting. I've seen folks in online chronic pain forums say they don't think they can go on living with the pain. (If you need help, call the 988 Suicide and Crisis Lifeline at 988, text the Crisis Text Line at 741741, or go to 988lifeline.org.)

DIFFERENT ANSWERS

For this book, I asked dozens of others who have chronic pain to give their best definition of it. Here's a representative sample of the responses:

"The medical definition misses the bigger picture. There's not only the physical component, but there's an emotional and spiritual factor that gets dampened the longer the pain continues. Chronic pain is almost a whole life experience." — Susan

"Life-altering pain that forces you to change who you are." — Mindi

"I think chronic pain is any discomfort that you live with that is constant and that your body tries to adapt to. The length of time is less important than the level of pain." — Roz

"I think chronic pain should be measured day-by-day. I have pain every day, but I don't have pain all day. I feel lucky in that. But the pain is still chronic. I know that six months from now, I will have pain." — Brad

"Chronic pain is different for different people, but the best thing I can say is that it is a constant pain that is so bad, it becomes a constant focus and makes it difficult to do even ordinary activities." — Jim

"I define chronic pain as the pain that sticks around with me all the time. It's like the weather. It'll be there tomorrow. It'll be there next month. It'll be there next year. I think limiting it to a certain number of months doesn't really accomplish much." — Mark

I asked the same question on a Facebook chronic pain support group. Here is a vivid answer:

"Chronic pain = hell on earth. Pain every day. It effects every aspect of your life. Makes you feel crazy. And it never goes away."

The takeaway from these responses: Chronic pain is far more than pain that lasts for greater than three to six months. It affects everything we sufferers do. It intrudes on our lives. It consumes the core of our being, our sense of self, our identity.

It that hyperbole? Talk with enough chronic pain sufferers and you'll hear stories of lives interrupted, relationships fractured, and potential lost.

"Talk with enough chronic pain sufferers and you'll hear stories of lives interrupted, relationships fractured, and potential lost."

HIGH IMPACT PAIN

In an effort to better capture the reality of chronic pain, researchers developed the concept of what's clunkily called "high impact chronic pain" (HICP). (I desperately want to pronounce that "hiccup.")

According to a study by the National Center for Complementary and Integrative Health's (NCCIH) Division of Intramural Research and collaborating institutions:

> *[HICP is] pain that has lasted three months or longer and is accompanied by at least one major activity restriction, such as being unable to work outside the home, go to school, or do household chores.*

The study of HICP by the NCCIH showed some dramatic results:

> *About 83% of people with High Impact Chronic Pain were unable to work for a living, and one-third had difficulty with self-care activities such as washing themselves and getting dressed.*

> *Compared to people with chronic pain without … limitations, those with [HICP] had higher levels of anxiety, depression, fatigue, and cognitive difficulty. They [reported] more severe pain, worse health, and higher healthcare use.*

HICP is widespread. According to the Center for Disease Control and Prevention (CDC), in 2023:

> *8.5% of adults had chronic pain that frequently limited life or work activities (referred to as high impact chronic pain) in the past three months. American*

Indian and Alaska Native non-Hispanic adults were significantly more likely to have chronic pain (30.7%) compared with Asian non-Hispanic (11.8%) and Hispanic (17.1%) adults.

LIFE DERAILED

I fall into the HICP category, with my condition causing my life to derail.

At age 53, I had to retire early and go on federal disability (see chapter 4). I lost the working life that was at the core of my identity.

I am mobility impaired. I walk with a cane for short distances and use a wheelchair for longer ones. It's hard to get out and enjoy life.

I've struggled with depression (see chapter 10) and anxiety, which often accompany chronic pain.

My relationships have been affected. My wife was forced into being a caregiver (see chapter 24). She handles that with grace, and I am grateful to her.

Still, carving out the category of HICP is not enough to describe the depth of my pain and that of others I've interviewed and read about.

There's at least one more competing definition of chronic pain. Some doctors see chronic pain as simply that which endures absent of original injury, after physical damage has supposedly healed. For example, according to the Institute for Chronic Pain:

There is a tendency among patients and some healthcare providers to continue to see the pain as a symptom of the underlying health condition that started it. They think of chronic pain as simply the long-lasting pain of an injury or illness that hasn't yet healed.

This line of thinking leads to getting a lot of healthcare. Surgeries, injections, and narcotic pain medications are common attempts to reduce pain by focusing on the underlying condition that started the pain. The typical chronic pain patient has had any number of such procedures and therapies.

… Studies of healthcare expenditures show that in the last twenty years the rates of pain-related surgeries, injections, and narcotic pain medications are at an all-time high. At the same time, applications for pain-related disability are also at an all-time high. Obviously, these procedures and therapies don't work so well.

Chronic pain has two characteristics that are different from acute pain. First, chronic pain lasts longer than six months. Second, and most importantly, chronic pain is pain that occurs in addition to the pain of the original health condition. In fact, the original, underlying condition may or may not have healed. It doesn't really matter. Chronic pain is pain that has become independent of the underlying injury or illness that started it all.

MY DEFINITION

"Chronic pain sucks."

What is the true definition of chronic pain? Let me venture my own:

Chronic pain sucks. It goes on long past the normal time for healing, disrupting sufferers' lives and making it hard to focus on anything else. It impacts relationships, mobility, and work. It is affected by emotions — and emotions affect it. Living with it requires not just physical treatments but social, psychological, and occupational ones as well. For sufferers, chronic pain endures, entraps, and seems endless.

What do you think? If you are a chronic pain sufferer, have I captured your experience? Does that make sense?

TOWARD A COMMON UNDERSTANDING

It is difficult to describe chronic pain if we do not have a common understanding to guide us.

It's essential that we spread a more precise definition of chronic pain and the impact it has on sufferers. It gets confusing when we sufferers, healthcare providers, media members, and policymakers can't agree on a meaning that truly captures the experience of chronic pain.

We need a mutual definition to help the tens of millions of Americans out there struggling to live, love, and earn a livelihood.

Let's get to work.

14

What Chronic Pain Feels Like

*Never-ending aches, stabs, zaps, and being stepped on
by an elephant in stilettos*

People like me who are in chronic pain struggle to be seen, heard, and understood.

We often lack the words to describe what we go through daily to family, friends, doctors, physical therapists, policymakers, and others.

I've taken a stab at it throughout this book; for example, I've likened it to being a sponge dipped in acid, about as vividly as I can to describe my own experience.

"For me, it feels like [I've been] run over by a car, then thrown off a cliff."

But what do others feel?

As part of researching for this book, I've uncovered some other answers to what chronic pain really feels like.

CHRONIC PAIN CHRONICLES

Here are insightful descriptions of pain drawn from the r/ChronicPain Reddit group (lightly edited for spelling, grammar, punctuation, length, and clarity):

My stomach feels like a bag full of Tabasco and broken glass mixed with boiling oil that's being drilled into [me] all day long.

Feels like you are a middle school kid who gets bullied and beaten up every day.

My favorite analogy is that my body feels like when you [crumple] up a shirt and shove it in the corner of a suitcase. [I] literally cannot explain what that means but it makes perfect sense in my head. Just … crumpled.

I get zaps of pain that feel like electric shocks or bee stings. In fact, a wasp stung my foot the other day and it took me a moment to realize it was a wasp, and not my normal pain. Lol.

I told my doctor once that it feels like my bones are made of glass and my muscles and nerves are being held taut over their sharp framework.

Like the world's worst hangover mixed with COVID.

My lower back feels like I worked a double [shift] as a server on Mother's Day.

I describe [most of my pain] as like being randomly attacked by knife-wielding ghosts. Occasionally the pain is very intense, blunt, and feels like it's in my bones. In this case, I call it ghosts [wielding] golf clubs [or] tire irons.

Sharp, stabbing pain. When I cough, sneeze, or orgasm, I have to brace myself. So, I avoid having a cold, flu, and sex…lol. And laughing. If I laugh really hard, I feel like passing out.

"I feel like my ribs are a tight corset to my torso [and] every breath I take is knives stabbing between my ribs."

Some days it's like a deep ache, which is more frustrating than debilitating. Other days it feels like my whole upper body has been battered for hours by Mike Tyson in his prime.

In my most comfortable resting state: getting slapped in the nuts every 20–30 seconds. While on my feet cooking or in the shower: Getting slapped in the nuts every 5–10 seconds. While walking: Getting slapped in the nuts every 5–10 seconds while a demon cracks me across the thigh, knee, shin, ankle, and foot with five wooden baseball bats every time I take a step with my left leg.

Some parts [of my body] burn like searing onions. Some parts are boiled dry potatoes. The rest is an Eeyore of drizzling wet sawdust.

When I get a flare-up, I describe it [to others] as feeling like a spear rammed through my back and out through my chest. I don't bother describing the rest of it after that, as the person asking is usually not that interested.

At its apex, the pain feels like someone [has placed] a 360° vise around my rib cage, crushing my lungs [and making] it hard to breathe deeply without pain. If I lie down, my voice even sounds like I'm being crushed.

Like I've run a 1,000 km marathon uphill in July in Arizona with a backpack of boulders on my back. If I stop and rest, I'm pretty much staying in that spot for the next 12 hours; if I keep going, my hearing starts going and my vision is turning black and I start shaking with every step. It's hell on earth.

I call the pain in my hips 'the chicken wing feeling' because it feels like what pulling apart a chicken wing looks like.

My knees feel like old, rusty hinges. Sometimes they grind. Sometimes they creak. Sometimes they are stiff. Sometimes they give out. If I move too fast or the wrong way? Uh, oh: bad mojo.

I feel like I've been giving a piggyback ride to someone who has his or her knees [digging] into my back at all times.

[My] muscles feel like they are a dishrag being wrung out tightly without a release.

> *"It feels like all the nerves/veins/arteries/muscles in my jugular area are being squeezed and pulled by King Kong."*

My migraines usually feel like someone or something is squeezing my temples and my eyes are full of chlorine.

Like you took a nerve and smashed it under a hydraulic press, or like I just ate 2,000 boxes of free Chinese food from some alleyway.

Feels like I've been stepped on by an elephant walking in stilettos.

WHAT I HEAR

It's common for chronic pain sufferers to be dismissed. It's easy to say that they engage in hyperbole. Sometimes the main response to such descriptions is, "Man up, and get over it."

But that's not what's going on in the Reddit chronic pain group and other spaces where sufferers gather to share and commiserate.

I hear real people in pain who are fighting to make others understand how they feel with whatever, and however imperfect, metaphors they can think of.

I hear hurt people desperate to be heard, healed, and held.

I hear cries for help.

104

15

It's 'All in Your Head'

*Understanding how the brain processes
pain can help cure it*

I admit I was pissed.

A couple of years ago, I took a course on chronic pain offered by the county I live in near Philadelphia. It promised to teach me how to better cope with the hurt I feel from a rare genetic disease that causes me to constantly ache from head to toe, with daily stabs in places like my lower back, shoulders, and feet.

The class textbook was called *Living a Healthy Life with Chronic Pain* by a host of pain experts from such places as Stanford University, Memorial University in Newfoundland, Canada, and the University of Missouri.

> *"The ... textbook contained the idea that offended me."*

The first chapter of the textbook contained the idea that offended me:

> *Let's say you just stubbed your toe. Within nanoseconds, the nerve endings in your toe that respond to pressure send a pattern of nerve impulses along the 'nerve highway' — the nerves in your toe, foot, leg, buttock and up to the spinal cord in your back. The spinal cord is like a superhighway of nerves that connect to your brain. It's your brain that asks: 'How dangerous is this really?' It's only when the brain thinks the pattern of nerve impulses are dangerous that pain is felt. In other words, pain is not in your toe, although it sure feels like that. Pain is produced by your brain to tell you and your body to take action. Because this is so important, it bears repeating: All pain is 100% in the brain.*

That last part — "All pain is 100% in the brain" — hit me wrong. I got angry. It sounded to me very much like what chronic pain sufferers hate being told: "The pain is all in your head."

Basics of PRT

Pain Reprocessing Therapy
(PRT) seeks to teach the brain
new tricks to relieve chronic
pain. According to its website:

*PRT is a system of psy-
chological techniques that
retrains the brain to interpret and respond to signals
from the body properly,
subsequently breaking the
cycle of chronic pain.*

PRT has five main
components:

1. **Education about the
   brain origins and
   reversibility of pain**
2. **Gathering and
   reinforcing personalized
   evidence for the brain
   origins and reversibility
   of pain**
3. **Attending to and
   appraising pain
   sensations through
   a lens of safety**
4. **Addressing other
   emotional threats**
5. **Gravitating to positive
   feelings and sensations.**

I am not endorsing PRT. I
have not done it and it can be
controversial and expensive.
Still, it has helped some (see
Pain Profile: Cured by Brain
Retraining).

That often means the person who says it, sometimes
a doctor, thinks that a patient's pain is false, entirely
made up, purely psychological rather than physical,
as though that makes it any less real.

WOMEN TEND TO BE DISMISSED

Women tend to be told this a lot, especially when a
doctor — often male — can't find a physical reason
for pain. They are dismissed as hysterical, as exaggerating, as too sensitive (see chapter 19).

A study cited in the *Proceedings of the National
Academy of Sciences* reinforces this idea:

*Physicians treat men and women differently when
it comes to pain. ... The analysis found that, when
first arriving at hospital, women were 10% less
likely than men to have a recorded pain score — a
number from 1 to 10, given by the patient, that
helps to inform physicians about the severity of
pain. After the initial assessment, women waited
an average of 30 minutes longer than men to see a
physician and were less likely than men to receive
pain medication.*

TRUE OR FALSE?

The idea that pain is "all in your head" and, therefore, not legitimate is false.

In his book *The Way Out: A Revolutionary,
Scientifically Proven Approach to Healing Chronic
Pain* (written with Alon Ziv) Alan Gordon, LCSW,
the founder of the Pain Psychology Center in
Beverly Hills, California, observes:

*Pain is pain, and it is always real. And because
all pain is processed in the brain, our brains have
extraordinary power to affect where, when, and
how much pain we experience.*

Once I read more about pain being processed in the

brain, I understood that in another sense, it's true that pain is all in your head.

Pain takes place in the brain — therefore, the head. Signals from nerves throughout the body travel through the spinal cord to the brain, where they are interpreted.

Sometimes this is simple. We experience a problem somewhere. We may need a Band-Aid, an ibuprofen, or, in worst cases, an emergency department trip.

Sometimes, though, the brain plays tricks.

For instance, while writing this essay just now, I felt something touch my left hand between the thumb and index finger. I looked down. Just for a split second, I "saw" a big black spider crawling on my skin. Then, almost immediately, I realized it was just a dark-blue-and-black piece of twine on a zipper on my shorts. I swear it happened. For that instant, my brain had convinced me I was under attack, and I experienced a fight, flight, freeze response.

Thanks for lying to me, brain.

CEREBRAL STORYTELLER

Why does something like this happen? As any fiction lover knows, the brain is incredibly good at creating stories, including reasons for pain.

The brain tries to assign meaning to the sensations we feel. It seeks an explanation. It tells tales, even if they aren't true. My brother calls the brain's ability to mislead us M.S.U. — "making shit up."

We tend to trust our thoughts, thinking we are totally in touch with reality. After all, what can we rely on if not our own brains?

But that is too simplistic an idea. We are all aware of how two people can see the world completely differently (say, politics, marriage, or sports fandom). Despite having similar brains in common, each of us has our own experiences, emotions, and expectations.

BRAIN CHANGE

Again, the brain plays tricks. This is due to neuroplasticity, which means the brain processes pain not just on physical sensation, but on memory, other sensory input, experience, and expectation (see Foreword).

Gordon explains:

'Neuroplasticity' refers to the brain's ability to learn and change. It's something that humans are uniquely good at. But when the brain learns and changes in response to pain, it can become chronic. That's [called] neuroplastic pain.

There's no consensus about how exactly pain is interpreted in the brain. There appears to be overlap between the parts of the brain that process pain signals and the parts of the brain that process emotions. Further studies, as they say, are needed.

However, according to Gordon:

"We've helped people overcome every form of pain imaginable."

Over the past decade, thousands of fMRI studies have been done on different aspects of pain. While there is still a lot to learn, we've made two major discoveries. First, it's become clear that chronic pain is completely different from short-term pain. It acts differently, responds to treatment differently, and even involves different parts of the brain. … Second, pain is much more complicated than we originally thought. There isn't just one 'pain center' of the brain; fMRI studies have found that multiple areas of the brain are associated with pain. And when I say 'multiple,' I mean multiple."

To help his patients, Gordon and colleagues developed a technique called Pain Reprocessing Therapy (PRT) (see sidebar) to essentially retrain the brain to think about pain differently. Though controversial among some, believers say it takes advantage of the brain's ability to form new neural pathways to break entrenched pain patterns and replace them with new ones.

As for results, Gordon reports in his book:

Over the years, we've refined our techniques into a consistently effective system … and we've helped people overcome every form of pain imaginable.

GIVE AND TAKE

PRT teaches the brain to reduce the worry, fear, and dread patients feel in favor of more neutral emotions. It takes conditioned responses in the brain and breaks their hold (see Pain Profile: Cured by Brain Retraining).

Over time and with a lot of work, Gordon has seen people with significant pain get better:

In each case, patients experience physical symptoms, but physical treatments don't help. By targeting the brain instead of the body, patients can finally get relief from their pain.

When it comes to curing — or at least easing — chronic pain, it is clear that understanding chronic pain is all in your head can help sufferers cope with it.

Gordon concludes, "If your brain can give you pain, it can also take it away."

PAIN PROFILE

Pain Poser

A lifelong chronic pain sufferer finds relief on stage

Roz Potenza loves to act.

The 65-year-old, who lives in the "steamy, humid" Tampa Bay, Florida, area is most at home on stage as a professional performer, but Potenza does another kind of acting: pretending that she's not in chronic pain. She explains:

> *I do live theater. I was in a long-running show called* Shear Madness. *It required me to be onstage for the entire 2 1/2 hours. The pain was excruciating at times, cutting across my lower back, my neck — and even my knee joined the party.*

> *Some days, though, I feel like a pain poser. I do. I think there are others who have it so much worse with painful diseases and conditions. It's a strange comparison thing.*

"The pain was excruciating at times."

WHERE IT HURTS

The New Jersey native who lives with her husband of more than 30 years and two Great Danes hurts throughout her entire body, something to which many seniors can relate.

> *My chronic pain starts in my neck and shoulders. I feel it most in my left shoulder around the shoulder blade, but it often shifts sides. The pain can be dull under the bony blade or all-encompassing and run across both shoulders. It also runs up my neck, giving me headaches. I now have what I refer to as a 'hot spot,' a section to the left of my lower neck and shoulder that hurts all the time. The pain feels like my skin is burning. Touching it hurts.*

She can manage her pain reasonably well and it doesn't confine her most of the time, so Potenza doesn't tell people about it unless they are "really" close to her.

People want to challenge you or one-up you. Oh, you have that? I have it so much worse.' We all do each other a disservice when we do this to each other. My pain is mine alone. I cannot compare it to others. Each one of us has a unique experience, whether it stems from a similar situation or not. I'm not worried about being judged, but I am aware of stigmas surrounding chronic pain and the meds that go with it.

If asked, Potenza is truthful about her pain, saying, "Some folks get it, and some don't. I can't do anything about that. Most of my friends and some family members don't know."

LONG-TERM HURT

Potenza's pain ranges back to age 12 when she had the first in a series of car accidents.

My mother's car was T-boned, and I was ejected from the vehicle. After that, I was involved in another six car accidents ranging from minor fender benders to some rather nasty stuff like being rear-ended by a school bus, and another time going head-on into a car that ran a stop sign. I had severe whiplash from the first accident, and it gradually got worse from the others, but what did that mean? To me, 'pain' was just a word. Doctors didn't do much except to give me a foam cervical collar. Stupid treatment.

In her late teens, Potenza began riding horses. She recalls:

I have been thrown off of them in every direction one can imagine. I broke thoroughbreds for a living for about three years until I had to stop. I loved barrel racing my quarter horse. Repeatedly banging my knees on the barrels caused pain that I suffer from still.

As she grew into adulthood, pain problems piled on. In her late 20s, Potenza developed cystic ovaries and had a large uterine mass that kept coming back.

Then, when she hit 50, Potenza was diagnosed with breast cancer.

Post-treatment, I was put on Tamoxifen theoretically to keep the cancer from coming back. It caused great muscle and joint pain. After eight years, they said it wasn't helping me and to stop taking it, but the damage was done.

Regardless of the setbacks, Potenza has kept searching for pain relief.

I've had many cortisone shots in my neck and knees. I have done tons of physical therapy and massage therapies. I've gotten some relief using medical marijuana in oil form. I've tried a pain patch recently, but it causes me horrible pain due to my skin sensitivity. It felt like a thousand red ants on my skin. I also own every pain-relief device known to man, for back pain: rollers, pins, electronic thumping guns, and massage machines with and without heat options. I even had a neck stretcher that inflated. It was meant to take the pressure of your head off your neck. Using it, I looked like something out of a sci-fi movie.

HANGING IN THERE

Despite her pain, Potenza still works.

I am a professional actress, and my husband and I own a small retail jewelry shop. I manage an online presence and do pearl restringing. It's a lot on my neck to look down for hours so I have to add time to each job so I can take breaks when the pain becomes too much to bear. I also do costume work but again, the position one needs to sustain is head down over a sewing machine or project, so I don't take big jobs anymore. For fun, I write.

Potenza gets the most relief on stage.

Perhaps it was because I was engaged with the text and the audience. I love performing and find it very invigorating. My pain threshold gets worse as the day goes into night. There have been many times doing Shear Madness *when I either had to sit down or excuse myself briefly during rehearsals so that I could take something to relieve my pain or, at least, tamp it down. But by the end of the show's run, my body got into a rhythm with it as well.*

> "*I looked like something out of a sci-fi movie.*"

Potenza concludes: "I get great satisfaction from performance. One can almost forget about the pain when engaged onstage."

KEYS TO COPING

Potenza says her pain journey taught her lessons on how to take care of herself. She believes these are the keys to coping with the emotions of chronic pain:

Eating right

I try to eat healthy and get some sunshine. Vitamin D is beneficial. I've started seeing a physician who is an osteopath. She has put me on a hefty dose of supplements that help my body feel better and therefore able to deal with my pain better. I am a firm believer in a healthy mind and healthy body. It doesn't work all the time, but overall, it helps me navigate my daily pain.

Healthy grieving

I have gone through a state of mourning about the 'old me,' and I have let that go. I have come to accept where I am in my life. I think we might need to go through a grief period. It's healthy to acknowledge that you aren't the same person you were. If you stay mired in that state, then you need to talk to someone. I call this my new normal, although after so many years, it's not so new.

Acceptance

I do accept that this is who I am now. I'm still a touch in denial because I can manage to do almost everything I need to do. I am aware that planning things helps. I have a different approach to how I achieve my goals now.

Gratitude

I try to feel grateful every day. I try. I don't always achieve it. On days when gratitude stays just out of reach, I practice mindfulness. What do I mean by that? I mean that I'm not always happy about certain things, but I'm mindful that it could be worse. It doesn't make things hurt less, but it makes me take a breath.

Self-compassion

You have to love yourself. Self-loathing is a sure trip to being worse off. I don't always have a happy attitude, especially on bad pain days, but I do my best to say tomorrow will be better. If it isn't, then I push to the next day. It's not easy. I keep moving and I feel lucky to be able to do so. I know so many who can't.

16

Cruel Loneliness

*A survey offers a disturbing portrait of
what it's like to live with pain*

Here's the thing you aren't told about living in chronic pain: It's lonely as hell.

My pain is isolating. It's like being trapped in solitary in a prison with only my own thoughts for company. There's an eerie sense of being cut off from the general population, all by myself. No matter how hard I try to explain what my experience is like to others, there's still a fundamental disconnect.

In this sense, I am like the vast majority of chronic pain sufferers, according to a 2025 survey by the U.S. Pain Foundation (see Sources of Solace).

Among other results, the survey of nearly 2,100 self-selected people living with chronic pain found that their pain is deeply lonely, long-lived, misunderstood, and stigmatized. As depressing as that sounds, understanding pain sufferers' struggles better is a key to helping them find relief.

> *"Pain isolates sufferers."*

LIVING IN ISOLATION

Pain isolates sufferers socially and robs them of the relationships that make life so rich, including love and romance. Notice the huge majority of sufferers who reported similar experiences in the survey:

- 90% missed social events in the past year due to their pain.

- 79% said their pain makes it difficult to spend time with family or friends.

- 73% felt socially isolated or misunderstood.

- 70% said their romantic relationships were significantly impacted.

- 65% reported difficulty communicating with loved ones about their pain.

- Only 28% said their family and friends are very supportive.

Nicole Hemmenway, the CEO of the U.S. Pain Foundation, tells me:

"Nine out of 10 sufferers have lived with pain for more than five years."

Chronic pain doesn't just affect the body — it can quietly unravel our relationships, our routines, even our sense of self. What this survey confirms — and what we hear every day — is that isolation itself becomes its own kind of pain: quiet, devastating, and deeply real. It means missing out on milestones, being misunderstood by loved ones, and feeling invisible and left behind in a world that keeps moving forward.

LONG-LIVED PAIN

By definition, chronic pain is enduring, but it's eye-opening how long sufferers deal with it. Once pain becomes chronic, it's notoriously difficult to remedy.

The survey, titled *Behind the Numbers: What It Really Means to Live With Chronic Pain* and released to coincide with Pain Awareness Month in September 2025, showed that about nine out of 10 sufferers have lived with pain for more than five years. Worse yet, almost one-third have lived in pain for more than a quarter of a century.

It also takes a long time for sufferers to get a diagnosis. Only 15% were diagnosed within six months of their pain's beginning. A third waited one to five years, and 29% got a diagnosis after five years. Others never get a reason for their pain.

Finding a provider to help is difficult: "21% had seen more than 10 providers in search of answers. Another 32% had seen between 6 and 10 providers," according to the report. It goes on to say:

Younger respondents — especially those under 35 — were more likely to report waiting three or more years for a diagnosis. This suggests systemic dismissal of younger people's pain, lack of access to specialists early on, or the bias that pain in youth or young adulthood is 'psychosomatic' or temporary.

Adults who were 55 and older were more likely to receive a diagnosis within a year of symptom onset, possibly reflecting more-frequent health care interactions, higher likelihood of belief from providers, or more obvious physical correlations with aging.

Even after years of seeking answers, many individuals continue to live with unexplained symptoms and a sense that something important has been over-looked. In fact, 38% of respondents — even those with a diagnosis — or their providers believe they still have undiagnosed conditions.

The implication is that large swaths of Americans endure significant pain for a remarkably long time. Despite the painful statistics, pain is relatively low on the national public health agenda.

PAIN IS COMPLICATED

One of the biggest challenges of coping with chronic pain is how complex it is. It often goes with other comorbidities (other conditions).

"Respondents reported an average of 10 distinct diagnoses per person. Conditions like back pain (64%), arthritis (53%), neuropathic or nerve pain (48%), osteoarthritis (42%), and fibromyalgia (37%) were among the most reported," said the survey results.

Further, it's hard to pin down pain. According to the report, a significant majority of sufferers have overlapping kinds of pain:

- 84% of those with inflammatory pain also had musculoskeletal pain.

- 83% of those with nociceptive (due to injury or tissue damage) pain also had neuropathic pain.

- 79% of those with musculoskeletal pain also had neuropathic pain.

"These patterns highlight the inadequacy of 'one-size-fits-all' care. Pain is not just felt in the nerves, joints, or tissues — it often spans all of these," concluded the report.

MENTAL TOLL

Pain also takes an intense emotional toll on sufferers. Nearly three-quarters reported a significant impact on their mental and emotional health. A similar percentage felt socially isolated or misunderstood. Exactly half said they lacked emotional support from others.

Chronic pain has a big impact on sufferers, severely limiting their lives:

- 93% said pain significantly limited physical activity or hobbies.

- 79% struggled with household chores.

117

- 76% reported serious sleep disruption.

- 76% missed work or school regularly.

- 74% said pain significantly interfered with employment or job performance.

- 61% were unable to care for children or dependents due to pain.

Pain hits some groups particularly hard:

Women often reported higher social and emotional impact across all ages in many categories. Nonbinary or gender-diverse respondents reported the greatest emotional burden—83% said their mental health was significantly affected. Adults between the ages of 35 and 64 experienced the most disruption to employment, relationships, and household chores. Adults who were 50 and older continued to face physical limitations, sleep disruptions, and challenges with household chores.

"61% ... experienced stigmatization."

THE STIGMA OF PAIN

I've written the stigma of pain (see chapter 33). The report reinforces that.

- 79% believe that stigma around chronic pain and its treatments is a major barrier to improving pain-related policies.

- 61% of sufferers have experienced stigmatization from providers or pharmacies related to opioid prescriptions.

- 21% are concerned about using medical cannabis or CBD for pain management because of associated stigma.

"Stigma was an all-too-common experience for respondents," the report's authors wrote. "Whether related to their condition or the treatments they use, individuals experienced stigma from a range of sources: friends, employers, family members, and even health care providers."

Stigma caused sufferers to be called "drug seeking," "difficult," and "dramatic."

"Such judgment reinforces isolation, discouraging individuals from advocating for the care they need or openly sharing their realities," the report said. The survey results further showed:

[M]ore care did not always mean better care. Among those with frequent appointments, 21% still felt 'not at all understood' by their providers, a similar rate as those seeing the doctor less frequently — highlighting persistent gaps in provider empathy, communication, and trust. Only 12% felt their providers fully understood their pain; 60% said others (medical and non-medical) don't understand at all. Only 3% felt very well understood.

THE BOTTOM LINE

This all sounds very depressing, and as a pain sufferer I can testify to how chronic pain can make one feel down. No rose-tinted glasses can put a cheery face on pain.

But we sufferers are not without hope. The intent of the survey is to show the rest of the world the reality of chronic pain, not sugarcoat it. Only by spreading the truth about pain — to the public and policymakers — can things start to change.

Comments U.S. Pain Foundation CEO Nicole Hemmenway:

The findings are sobering — and they should be. But within them is a powerful call to action that can no longer be ignored. What gives me hope is the strength and honesty of the respondents. By speaking up, they're breaking through the silence that has surrounded chronic pain for too long. Recognition is the first step — and with it, we can push for meaningful change in policy, healthcare, and society.

Remember, behind those stats are real people who have serious challenges in life. Start by showing us compassion and helping us feel less isolated.

Hemmenway concludes, "And to every person living with pain: we see you, we hear you, we recognize your experience, and you are not alone."

Pain Points

"Being seen and heard is incredibly helpful. There is a clear distinction between pity and compassion. Pity isolates and separates those who offer it from the recipient. Compassion connects the two parties, thus alleviating some of the loneliness."
—Michele Cambardella

"Chronic pain builds a quiet, unspoken prison — one where the body's suffering is only deepened by the loneliness that grows in its shadow." —HIMA

"Since I retired in January, I'm here with my wife, who suffers from chronic pain, almost 24/7. I do what I can, but it still doesn't scratch that isolation itch." —Joel Everhart

Pain Points are comments on this essay as it appeared originally on Medium.com. They are solely the opinion of the commentators and do not necessarily reflect the views of the book author or publisher.

17

Alarming Advice

A prominent physician explains how enduring hurt really works

My father was a fount of wisdom, including this gem: "You can't make love with a toothache."

In his own crude way, he meant that it's impossible to feel joy when you are in pain, either acute or chronic.

"Acute pain is a good thing because it alerts us that there is something broken or damaged that needs to be fixed," says Andrea Furlan, MD, professor of medicine at the University of Toronto and author of *8 Steps to Conquer Chronic Pain: A Doctor's Guide to Lifelong Relief.* "The problem is chronic pain, which does not serve any purpose; it is just a horrible nuisance that steals people's joy. What motivates me is that I have helped thousands of people with chronic pain to regain their joy."

> *"Chronic pain, which does not serve any purpose, [is a] horrible nuisance."*

I can tell you: It is indeed difficult to make love or engage in any other life activity when in constant hurt. Chronic pain robs the joy of living from people like me, leaving us to cope with our conditions, often alone (see chapter 16). It is a disease distinct from acute pain, which resolves within weeks. Chronic pain terrorizes its sufferers.

But it does not need to be like that. There are many ways to relieve chronic pain — physical and psychological. Unfortunately, most physicians, with their focus on "curing" conditions, do a bad job of it.

Conditions that are chronic aren't easily cured. Most often, they are to be endured.

121

Dr. Furlan on Coping with Chronic Pain

Dr. Andrea Furlan's biggest lesson for sufferers is to learn about chronic pain.

"The first step is to get pain neuroscience education," she says. "I use the example of diabetes. If a person is diagnosed with diabetes, the first thing that needs to happen is to teach that person what diabetes is. He or she might have never heard of the pancreas and insulin, and what insulin does to blood sugars. Nowadays, however, there are different ways to 'manage' diabetes. There is no 'cure.' A person who has diabetes, understands what diabetes is, and uses the right tools to manage diabetes can have a pretty normal life. He or she can live longer, participate in sports, go to school, have a career, raise children, and grow older with joy in life. Chronic pain is the same way."

"Once the person understands chronic pain neuroscience, then it's time to discuss this with the doctors," she adds. "And maybe even teach the doctors about what nociplastic pain is and ask for treatments specifically tailored to that."

"Because chronic pain is different from acute pain, many people, including the medical professionals, do not know how to treat it," says Dr. Furlan. "They use the same tools for acute pain — medication, MRIs, surgery, shots, creams — to treat chronic pain, and, of course, they will not get the same results. Therefore, people with chronic pain spend years, even decades, trying interventions that do not work."

Based on her experience with thousands of patients, Dr. Furlan has insight into how best to deal with chronic pain (see sidebar).

HOW CHRONIC PAIN WORKS

Pain is the body's alarm system. If we are injured or diseased, the alarm goes off, telling us something is wrong.

Hit your thumb with a hammer and the pain shoots out. It's actually a complex system that carries pain signals to the brain, which immediately interprets how bad the threat is. This triggers a response, which ranges from saying "Ouch!" to writhing on the floor.

This system is useful in bringing attention to damage done to the body. It signals you should do something right now. It may call for a Band-Aid, stitches, or surgery to fix the problem. The hope is that the injury heals and leaves you none the worse for wear.

Pain, though, is a terrible indicator of what's really wrong. Research shows no close correlation between feeling pain and the severity or damage to the body. The brain decides the intensity of the pain based not only on the injury but on experience, expectations, and emotions (see Foreword).

A paper cut may hurt like hell, but the actual

damage to the body is minor. Generally, this kind of pain heals within hours, days, or weeks. At some point, *Bam!* We're well again and the pain has passed.

But sometimes the pain endures. It becomes chronic, defined as pain that lasts beyond normal healing time, perhaps up to six months or even longer.

Dr. Furlan points out that pain is part of life. Nobody is immune to it (except in the 2025 movie *Novocaine*). But medicine needs to stop treating chronic pain using the same methods that are used for acute pain. These are two completely different things. She believes a lot of resources are wasted, like MRIs, injections, and surgeries, that don't really address the underlying problem. Dr. Furlan says: "The medical profession is still not taught properly about chronic pain. In medical school and residency programs they are taught about how to alleviate acute pain. But they know very little about chronic pain and its mechanisms."

"So, what is chronic pain?" Dr. Furlan queries in an online video. "It's when pain becomes the disease. It's the disease of the pain system. It is when pain comes with an emotional distress, interference with daily life, and cannot be accounted for by any other chronic pain condition."

CHRONIC PAIN IS LIKE A BROKEN FIRE ALARM

Dr. Furlan explains how chronic pain works: Imagine pain as a fire alarm that starts to blare. What do you do? Most call the fire department, equivalent to standard medicine. The firemen show up and quash the flames — problem cured.

> *"[Chronic pain] is when pain becomes the disease."*

But what if there is no fire and the problem is with the alarm? It blares even if there is no smoke. Who do you call then? The fire department is unnecessary — there're no flames to put out. The problem is that the alarm is defective. It sends signals that something scary has happened, but there is really little danger.

In this case, you'd do better at solving the problem by calling the alarm company to request someone expert in fixing that system, not in putting out fires.

That's what Dr. Furlan does in her practice. She addresses the false alarms that come from the brain misinterpreting pain signals. The problem is not just the injury, but that the brain and nervous system have become sensitized to experience pain, even after the underlying damage has healed.

"So, when medical professionals can't fix the pain (because it is not acute pain) many just dismiss their patients' complaints," Dr. Furlan observes.

"Another way to think about pain [is as a] damaged laptop."

SWITCHING METAPHORS

Another way to think about pain is to switch metaphors from an alarm system to a damaged laptop computer. Dr. Furlan illustrates this by talking about the three basic kinds of pain — nociceptive, neuropathic, and nociplastic (also called neuroplastic):

Nociceptive is equivalent to a computer that is not working because a car ran over it and broke the monitor, hard drive, the keyboard. It is damaged and needs replacing or fixing. This would be similar to a pain from arthritis in a bad knee. To treat the nociceptive pain, you do knee replacement surgery.

Neuropathic pain (nerve pain) is equivalent to a computer without a cord connecting to the electrical outlet. The battery has no way to be recharged, the computer doesn't work because there is a physical problem, and the problem is that the cord is broken or damaged or has just disappeared.

Nociplastic [neuroplastic] pain means the computer looks perfect: nothing broken or damaged. The battery is charged. The monitor is fine. The computer might even turn on, but it shows a blue screen with white text that doesn't mean anything to you. You need to fix the software, maybe uninstall and reinstall some programs.

Nociplastic pain is the most common form of chronic pain. It is based in the brain's natural "neuroplasticity," its ability to learn new things and make new neural connections. The good news is that if the brain is causing chronic pain, neuroplasticity means it can also solve the problem.

It turns out that chronic pain really is, in some cases, all in your head (see chapter 15). Dr. Furlan is careful to say, though, that the pain is very real. It should not be dismissed as purely psychological and therefore, not genuine or worth a physician's time. We sufferers can tell you that our hurt can be felt deeply in our tissue and bones.

Dr. Furlan and colleagues like her specialize in solving the software problem, which means changing how sufferers understand, think, and behave regarding their chronic pain. This might involve pain education, influencing sufferers' thinking and behavior toward pain, or encouraging healthier lifestyle choices, such as a better diet.

"No medication will fix nociplastic pain," she adds. "Actually, the side effects could make things worse (fatigue, constipation, nausea, etc.)."

THE EMOTIONS OF CHRONIC PAIN

Chronic pain and emotions are closely intertwined. Each affects the other. We see it in people's experiences, and pain sufferers report that their moods can make pain better or worse.

Chronic pain dredges up deep emotions, the seven most common of which I write about in chapter 14. Dr. Furlan says people spend years or decades of their lives trying interventions that do not work, so they develop these emotions:

> *Fear. This is the main fuel of chronic pain. The more fearful people are, the worse pain they feel. They are fearful of their pain, fearful of moving (exercise), fearful of the medical doctors cutting their painkillers, and so on.*
>
> *Anger. People feel anger at someone who was to blame for their accident. Or they blame the healthcare system for not helping them. They blame their family for not understanding them. They blame themselves for not having energy to do the exercises, lose weight, and take care of themselves.*
>
> *Despair. They feel hopeless. They think that they tried everything and so far, nothing has worked.*
>
> *Loneliness. Many people had to stop working or going to social functions due to pain. They lost their friends, connections with other people, coworkers, school, hobbies, travel.*
>
> *Worry. They worry about their future, what will happen to them, how will they take care of themselves when they get older. And they wonder: Could this condition get worse?*

POWERFUL METAPHORS

Thinking of chronic pain as a defective fire alarm or buggy computer software can help sufferers better understand how it can be addressed. Focusing on how the brain interprets pain signals is the pathway to relief. Expert physicians like Dr. Furlan can lead the way.

Interviewing Dr. Furlan and other chronic pain experts and sufferers has led me to realize that my pain is not to be feared. It's a natural part of the brain and the body, which can get stuck in a pain feedback loop, becoming chronic and reinforcing the hurt I feel throughout my body.

My pain is real but it is affected by how I think about my condition.

It's taught me I can make love even with my aches.

Sorry, Dad. You were wrong.

18

Conflated Crises

*Desperate chronic hurt sufferers are
caught between two health epidemics*

I felt like a criminal.

As I got out of my blue Chrysler PT Cruiser, I spotted cameras trained on
the parking lot. It occurred to me that they were there to spot suspicious drug
seekers.

Inside a nondescript medical building in Knoxville,
Tennessee, just off I-40, I entered the waiting room
of the pain clinic. The crowd, as my father would say,
"looked rough around the edges." I checked in with
the receptionist, who gave me a "seen it all, don't mess
with me" look.

*"I had a creepy
feeling."*

I knew the clinic was reputable, unlike the local pill mills that at the time gave
out prescriptions for opioids like Halloween candy. I was referred to it by my
trusted primary care physician. It wasn't seedy, just austere. Still, I had a creepy
feeling.

In a few minutes, I was called back to see the pain doctor. He quizzed me about
my chronic pain. I told him I suffer from a rare genetic disease that causes joints
to deform and degenerate over time. I was in my late 40s and had put a lot of
wear and tear on my body. I explained I'd had joint replacements and was in
chronic pain from head to toe.

I'd been on painkillers for decades, prescribed first by my orthopedist, then by
my primary care doctor. Back then, I took three 80-milligram OxyContin pills
(the largest dose sold by pharmaceutical manufacturer Purdue Pharma) plus
three acetaminophen-hydrocodone combination pills a day. I'd stayed on the
same strengths for years, but as my body broke down, I felt I needed more relief.

(I'm waffling by saying "I felt" because there is no objective way to measure whether more pain medication is necessary. Each pain sufferer's situation is unique. It comes down to his or her opinion of what's needed to feel relief.)

My primary care physician said he'd done all he could. He was limited by state and practice mandates that patients get only up to 100 morphine equivalent doses a day. If I wanted more, I needed to go to a specialized pain clinic.

To even get an appointment with the pain doc, I had to first pass muster with a psychologist at the clinic to confirm I wasn't just looking for a high. As I sat before him, I squirmed in my seat.

"Do you have a history of drug abuse?" the psychologist asked. "No," I answered. "Have you ever taken more medicine than directed?" Also, "No." "Do you think you have an addictive personality?" "No," again.

PASSING THE SCREENING

A week later, after I passed the screening, I got to see the MD specializing in pain, who could choose to prescribe something stronger than the Oxy and hydrocodone I took. Sitting in his office, I made my case. I said I had plateaued on the current doses. More medicine would ease my pain so I could continue to make a living and maintain a decent quality of life. I worked as an executive at a communications and marketing firm and had a wife and three daughters to provide for.

He thought for a moment. He looked at me skeptically. "Sorry," he said. "I don't think you are in enough pain to merit an increase. We're very careful prescribing opioids because of the addiction risk. There's nothing more we can do. We can take over prescribing your current medications. You'd have to undergo monthly drug testing. But we cannot go up on your prescriptions."

His statement was definitive. I recognized that no amount of persuasion could sway him. I walked out without the medical help I needed. Even though the pain clinic was legitimate, I had the gnawing sense that I was doing something shameful. Intimidated, chagrined, and discouraged, I stopped the process of changing physicians and returned to getting my pain medicine from my primary care doctor. Like many pain patients, I would have to tough out the pain on my current doses of drugs.

My experience was not unique. I had been caught in the collision of two massive public health issues — the opioid crisis and the chronic pain epidemic — with countless pain sufferers as collateral damage.

THE ROOTS OF WAR

The roots of this problem go back to the Richard Nixon administration.

On June 17, 1971, the president gave a speech in which he declared drug addiction "public enemy number 1." He added that, "In order to fight and defeat this enemy, it is necessary to wage a new all-out offensive."

"I had the gnawing sense that I was doing something shameful."

This launched the War on Drugs, an effort that's dragged on for more than half a century. The idea became deeply rooted in the public mind that we as a nation face a dire threat from illicit drugs and that we must slash their use without mercy.

Further, it demonized those using such street drugs as marijuana, cocaine, and heroin as dangers to themselves and others. Therefore, they need to be arrested and incarcerated, leading to a massive increase in the prison population. It created the image of all drug users as junkies, drug fiends, and addicts, all considered pejorative terms.

Fast forward to the '90s and the growing focus among authorities on pain in America. Indeed, major medical groups like the Veterans Administration labeled assessing a pain score as the "fifth vital sign" (after body temperature, blood pressure, pulse rate, and respiratory rate).

Enter Purdue Pharma. In 1996, it launched OxyContin, an extended-release version of the opioid oxycodone. According to its manufacturer, this was the miracle drug doctors were waiting for. Purdue marketed the pill as nonaddictive and safe to prescribe.

Physicians were primed because of the new focus on pain. A perfect storm of product and market occurred. Soon, doctors were giving patients pain pills for everything from joint replacement to wisdom teeth removal. And chronic pain.

Only later did people discover that Purdue lied. Extended-release OxyContin was highly addictive, particularly when crushed and ingested (say, by snorting the powder). Under the cover of the concern about pain, unscrupulous physicians prescribed millions of pills for those allegedly hurting. Abuse became rampant. The result was hundreds of thousands of deaths from opioid abuse and overdose from the '90s through today.

Scary stuff, but not the whole picture.

BACKLASH

The War on Drugs won some battles. Some physicians who ran pill mills went to jail. The Drug Enforcement Administration (DEA) corralled the supply of prescription opioids by cutting the amount manufacturers can make and distribute. Purdue Pharma, other drug manufacturers, and big pharmacy chains were sued and ended up on the hook for more than $50 billion in damages to individuals and states.

> *"A perfect storm of product and market occurred."*

Meanwhile, in 2016, the CDC issued guidelines aimed at cutting abuses and overdoses. Although not the CDC's intentions, doctors and others interpreted them as rules that put strict limits on the amount of opioids they could prescribe. The "guidelines" came off as restrictive, rigid, and regulatory.

In response, physicians, pharmacies, insurance companies, and state legislatures placed limits — like the 100 morphine equivalent doses I ran into — on the amount of relief pain patients could get.

But the restrictions produced a backlash. Legitimate pain patients complained that they could not get the medicine that made their lives bearable, that the guidelines did them more harm than good.

Under pressure, in 2022, the CDC rewrote and loosened its guidelines for prescribing opioids. According to the revised ones:

> *CDC recommends that persons with pain receive appropriate pain treatment, with careful consideration of the benefits and risks of all treatment options in the context of the patient's circumstances. Recommendations should not be applied as inflexible standards of care across patient populations.*

In other words, physicians should lighten up and treat pain patients individually, based on their unique circumstances. But these new guidelines were too little, too late. The message to doctors and the public had already been ingrained: Opioids bad, addictive, deadly.

Plus, beware: Doctors, healthcare workers, administrators, and pharmacists may be sued, lose their licenses, even go to jail if they overprescribe or overfill. No wonder they were — and are — scared silly.

That creates problems for pain sufferers. In online support groups of them on Facebook and Reddit, posters vent that they still can't get the drugs they need.

Doctors won't prescribe them, and pharmacies won't fill them out of fear of doing something wrong. I have seen enough folks complain on social media to know that the problem of medication restriction is real and widespread.

The stigma around opiates is so strong that those in pain are embarrassed to ask for and use them. Some will try anything to find relief but draw the line at taking drugs because of all the bad stories they have heard. I wonder how many pain sufferers would live better lives if they could get past the stigma and try appropriately prescribed opioid medication, which, despite its side effects, is still the most effective way to at once reduce severe pain. (Please note: Opioids have many side effects. Always obey warnings about operating heavy machinery and such. These drugs can be deadly.)

THE BATTLE TO WIPE OUT ABUSE

The opioid crisis unfolded in stages.

In the first phase, there was the flood of legally prescribed drugs to combat pain, which led to abuse by those who became addicted. In the second phase, as prescriptions were restricted, people turned to the streets for illegal drugs like heroin. The third stage has been the rise of the synthetic drug fentanyl, which is said to be up to 50 times more powerful than heroin and up to 100 times better at slashing pain than morphine.

Fentanyl has certainly been a scourge, but let's not forget it has many legitimate uses, like reducing pain after surgery, easing the suffering of late-stage cancer patients, and helping chronic pain patients.

It didn't help fentanyl's image that it was the villain in so many TV commercials during the 2024 election. The message was clear: Fentanyl is dangerous and those who use it are criminals. It has become a dirty word, code for all the crime, illegal immigration, and drug smuggling that some say threaten the American way of life.

It's true that fentanyl is often abused. Illegal fentanyl from Mexico has been infused into all kinds of counterfeit pills purported to be legit OxyContin, Percocet, and Xanax, for example. In fact, the DEA reports that in 2022 six out of 10 fake prescription pills contained potentially deadly doses of the drug. The result is about 150 people a day die from synthetic opioids.

I have defended fentanyl as being a killer in the wrong hands and a healer in the right ones (see chapter 27). Once the dangers of OxyContin were recognized, my primary care physician moved me from pills to fentanyl extended-release patches. I get a tiny amount of the drug through my skin — about 25 micrograms (0.000025 grams) per hour. I change the patch every three days.

Fentanyl doesn't get me high; it just takes the edge off the pain enough for me to function. If a tiny amount of it could kill, I'd be dead many times over.

(This is a good time to remind you I am not a doctor or healthcare professional. I am not qualified to endorse taking opioids or any other therapy for pain. Always enlist your physician's opinion before starting any treatment. Do not order any painkiller medicine or supplement from the internet or buy from friends or street sellers.)

FIGHTING THE WRONG WAR

So many physicians, policymakers, and others fail to realize that they are fighting the last war on drugs, not the current one. The problem with overdoses from *legally* prescribed medicine has largely been won. The CDC puts it this way: "Data shows that commonly prescribed opioids are no longer driving the overdose epidemic."

And, in terms of overall deaths from fentanyl and other drugs, recent trends show a promising (and unexpected) drop in overdoses (see chapter 35).

"I'd be dead many times over."

Reported *Stat* in 2025:

An estimated 80,391 people died of a drug overdose in the U.S. last year, marking the lowest total since 2019. The sum represents a roughly 27% decrease from 2023, according to the Centers for Disease Control and Prevention.

No one is sure quite why this is happening. It may be the enforcement or intervention is paying off and fewer people have become victims of drugs like fentanyl. The miracle cure Narcan is available in many more places. (Narcan, generic name naloxone, is now available over the counter without a prescription.) Or a grislier interpretation is that the people most likely to die from illegal drugs have and there simply aren't many left.

It's important to point out that it's *illegal* versions of opioids, rather than the legal ones, that now drive the War on Drugs.

Perhaps the problem is semantics. We talk about opioids as dangerous "drugs," but the truth is that in legitimate cases they should be simply called "medicine." There should not be shame for using them.

DEADLY CONSEQUENCES
Conflating (to bring together or blend) the pain epidemic and the opioid crisis has deadly consequences.

Television station WDRB in Louisville, Kentucky, reported:

> *On Sept. 18, 2017, Brent Slone texted this message to his wife: 'They denied script im done love you.' Thirty minutes later, he killed himself. According to the lawsuit filed against [a pain clinic] … Slone's suicide could have been prevented.*

(If you are struggling with thoughts of self-harm or suicide, call or text the Suicide & Crisis Lifeline at 988.)

In 2011, Slone was in a car accident that left him paralyzed and with other health problems. He went to a pain clinic in San Diego and received opioids. In 2018, he traveled to Louisville and contacted a local pain clinic to get his full slate of meds like those prescribed in California. The Kentucky clinic responded by cutting his prescription by 55% because paperwork from the San Diego prescriber was inadequate.

A jury found the Louisville-area pain clinic liable for $7 million because it refused to provide Slone with all his pain medications. WDRB.com doesn't give full details, but apparently Slone was in so much pain and desperate for relief that he decided to end his life.

It's certain that the Louisville-area clinic was being cautious because of federal guidelines, state restrictions, and the confluence of drugs and addiction with chronic pain. It's likely it feared repercussions if it made a mistake with Slone's prescriptions. So, it erred in the wrong direction and was ultimately held liable for Slone's death.

There's a lesson there: Continuing the War on Drugs by targeting patients in chronic pain has consequences. Confusing the problems of opiate abuse and chronic pain can be fatal.

UNTANGLING THE MESS
Chronic pain and drug abuse have become mixed up like a tangled skein of yarn. They are two separate things, but they've become entwined as though they are one issue.

The CDC cites a National Academies of Sciences report that describes the mix-up this way:

> *The ongoing opioid crisis lies at the intersection of two substantial public health challenges — reducing the burden of suffering from pain and containing the rising toll of the harms that can result from the use of opioid medications.*

The result is mass confusion among physicians, policymakers, and the public about how to help people in pain while preventing addiction and overdose deaths.

I understand that there is always a chance that someone will become addicted to prescription opioids. But in fact, researchers estimate odds of only 10% of that happening. I'm among the 90% that haven't become addicted despite my long history of using opioids.

"Continuing the War on Drugs by targeting patients in chronic pain has consequences."

Like a good little patient, I have always followed the directions for taking my medicine and have not abused them. Even though I have Narcan in the cabinet under my bathroom sink, I have never come close to needing it.

Our society doesn't stigmatize people taking statins to fend off heart problems. We don't demonize those who have broken legs and need casts. No one looks down on patients who have cancer and need chemo. In the same way, please don't judge those who are chronic pain sufferers and need medicine to cope.

It's time to untangle the two public health crises and see them as separate issues. We must deal with each one individually. Don't view those in chronic pain as drug seekers, addicts, and overdosers, but rather as legitimate patients. Let doctors and pharmacists do their jobs.

I use fentanyl. I am not a drug seeker. I am not a danger to others. I am not a criminal.

I'm simply a sufferer — one of many — who needs help.

Pain Points

"I work in a pain management practice. We care for both chronic pain sufferers and persons with substance use disorders. One issue on my end is having to jump through more and more hoops to prescribe opioids both with pharmacists and insurance companies [who ask] 'Why does your patient need this medication?!' Much of this relates to the ongoing War on Drugs as well as penalties the chain pharmacies are paying for their part in the original opioid crisis. Some are now going so far as to not stock opioids, so they don't have to deal with the issue. In my state the DEA regularly audits pharmacies. I have been using more buprenorphine (the active drug in Suboxone) to treat chronic pain because it has advantages over full opioids like oxycodone. One issue these patients encounter is the stigma at pharmacies when they fill their prescriptions. 'I [am] being treated like a drug addict!' I've lost count of the times I have said to people, 'Making me fill out a prior authorization every three months for someone's medications is not going to stop people from dying of fentanyl.'" —Janet Bebee

"Bringing chronic pain down a couple of notches is medicine. Those judging have no idea what people go through, until they face horrible pain." —Pearl Janz

"The way doctors treat you like an addict for asking to raise your dosage? It's because of people like me. I spent 16 years addicted to OxyContin and in my addiction, you can bet I drove doctors crazy trying to get my hands on it, lying and inventing stories in an effort to get it. I'm a direct part of the reason why people like my spouse and you have such a hard time getting what you need from doctors. I think about that every single day. If I could go back in time and change it, I would. I am so very sorry. I hope in the future doctors have a way of being able to effectively help people like you while still discouraging misuse." —Adriene Adams

Pain Points are comments on this essay as it appeared originally on Medium.com. They are solely the opinions of the commentators and do not necessarily reflect the views of the book author or publisher.

PAIN PROFILE

Rebelle's Revelation

A sufferer seeks solace by listening to her body

Lying in a pitch-black room with needles stuck in her body, Rebelle Summers had a revelation.

The 38-year-old digital nomad recalls her first acupuncture session a few years ago:

> "I hate needles, but I was at such a desperate point with my chronic pain that I was ready to try anything. I went to an acupuncture training school that came recommended for the quality of its students and its affordability. A lovely student and her supervisor led me into a clinical room. They had me lie down on my back while they explained everything they were going to do."

> "I was at such a desperate point with my chronic pain that I was ready to try anything."

After the student acupuncturist transformed her into a "human pincushion," Summers began to shiver. The practitioner gave her a foil blanket to keep her warm, turned off the lights, and left as the needles did their work. Summers remembers:

> I was alone in the pitch-black room with my thoughts. As I lay there with my eyes closed, an image of a newborn infant, scared and shaking, popped into my head. In that moment I realized that the baby was me, my defenseless little body, and that I, now as an adult, wanted to do everything I could to protect it. I felt tears trickling down my temples. My body finally relaxed. I had never experienced that kind of love and devotion toward myself. That one session transformed the entire trajectory of how I would approach my pain, leading with self-compassion first. I am my protector, and it is my job to give myself the best life possible.

137

FOREVER IN PAIN

Summers says she has experienced chronic pain "for as long as I can remember." She was diagnosed with endometriosis at age 14 and with fibromyalgia in her late twenties. She recalls:

"I resented my body for an extraordinarily long time."

But prior to those diagnoses I was chronically ill, practically from birth, and felt constantly worn down. Some of it may have been normal kid crud that became exacerbated due to living in a sensitive body, but I believe my home environment also contributed to the pain I was in and explained why I'd be so sick so often.

Two car accidents in her late teens compounded her health problems:

> *I resented my body for an extraordinarily long time. I blamed it for holding me back from career success, healthy relationships, and being a 'normal' person who could live life the way I wanted. I isolated frequently and perceived I was a burden to others. I masked the pain as much as possible. I even used it as a chip on my shoulder that motivated me to be extremely ambitious, which would begin the cycle of illness, and I would burn out again and again. But I didn't want people to suspect there might be something wrong with me. I didn't want to have to deal with people looking at me with pity, as if I were some pale, Dickensian orphan.*

Summers says her pain moves all over. Before she began taking care of herself, she felt a full-on body ache that she tried to repress and push through. Her occasional flare-ups typically burn.

> *And even on good days the pain has a bruising, tender quality to it. The achiness will mostly congregate around my scapulas up to my neck and in the arches of my feet or feel like a tight squeeze in my chest around my heart. The burning will show up in my quads, sometimes making it incredibly difficult to walk. The bruising sensation comes and goes but is more pronounced in my hips and abdomen but also doesn't discriminate and spreads all over.*

ON THE ROAD

Summers has worked on the road since 2021, when she was forced out of a rental house in Tucson, Arizona, because the owner wanted to move back in.

She has traveled the U.S., U.K., and Europe working as a freelance writer and audio engineer and producer. She says holding a standard 9-to-5 job wears down her body, so she gets sick often. Unfortunately, Summers is unable to get good insurance or benefits. She explains:

Due to my chronic conditions and how I need to live to make life manageable, I work freelance. This means I am chronically un- or underemployed and cannot easily find a permanent place to live. On top of that, I don't know where I want to be long term. As unfortunate as the beginnings of this chapter of my life have been, I've been given the opportunity to experience living elsewhere with all of the thrills and complications that come with that. So far, I have found that living outside the U.S. is much more accessible, affordable, and leisurely.

After realizing she needed to listen to her body, Summers finally made her chronic pain a priority. She "threw spaghetti at the wall" and worked with a variety of doctors, used medications, and invested in treatments such as cognitive behavioral therapy (CBT), internal family systems therapy (IFS), eye movement desensitization and reprocessing (EMDR), and mindfulness work.

She also collaborated with a naturopathic doctor and tried acupuncture, massage, and craniosacral work. She found that her body responded most positively to gentler "somatic processing modalities" through which she learned about different body systems and how to interpret and take action on messages they send. She also removed herself from relationships she believed worsened her pain.

I realized that my pain wasn't out to get me but was trying to communicate with me. It took awhile, but I was able to allow more compassion and grace for myself. This made it easier to decide whether certain pain needed a physical solution or emotional solution, or if I just needed to accept it for what it is. Remembering to rest has also been a game-changer for me.

As for relationships, Summers reports that her pain has been a "constant cloud" hanging over them:

There is the continuing bracing for outright dismissal or accusations of manipulation from folks due to the idea that pain and illness are only supposed to happen to people in later stages of life. There's also the equally offensive stance of believing my pain but perceiving and treating me with pity. The worst part of having chronic pain is not having enough people in my life who can hold space for how chronic pain inconsistently affects basic daily functions. People don't get that the pain's effect on me is only one aspect of who I am and how I experience my life.

"*Recognizing the function of pain altered my relationship to it.*"

PAIN THAT PROTECTS

Summers says her recognition that "the pain was not trying to hurt me but was actually trying to protect me" changed her life.

Recognizing the function of pain altered my relationship to it, to my body, and to how I approach life so that the pain and thereby I are moving through the world with more dignity. I gain a lot through self-examination and working to understand my pain and its function. Learning where it may have come from has helped me become more easeful, more discerning, and more assertive when it comes to my boundaries and limitations. I feel like I've always been a resilient and resourceful person, but my learning to have ease and find joy has created more balance in my life.

Overall, Summers has come to accept her pain. She recommends other pain suffers prioritize their needs as best and as much as they can, and learn what their bodies respond to.

For me, it began with acknowledging and reorienting my life around the basic signals my body would send me: feeling hungry, needing to use the restroom, being tired or energized. It may seem a little silly, but until I started doing that, I hadn't realized how much I was crossing my own body's boundaries by ignoring them or pushing them off to prioritize whatever I was working on or the people I was with. Living with chronic pain has meant needing to become friends with grief on a day-to-day basis.

Summers concludes:

Everyone's chronic pain story is different, each case its own fingerprint. What helps one person won't make a dent for another. But what affects each of us is the grief of not living the life we thought we would, of being denied the spaces we should easily access, and of not receiving adequate care. It can be daunting and frustrating not knowing how I'm going to physically feel each day when I wake up, but it also makes me more present so I'm living life less on autopilot and with more discernment and care.

19

Dissed and Dismissed

Because of bias, women have to work harder to get their pain taken seriously

Jana Barrett is a strength-and-conditioning coach, personal trainer, and "mobility alchemist" in Wellington, New Zealand.

She works with many clients, mostly women, in chronic pain, including one whose husband passed away from a heart attack.

"Within days, the whole left side of her body froze up and became extremely tense; she developed severe chronic pain that lasted for years," Barrett tells me.

The client worked with Barrett and a traditional Maori massage practitioner for women (Maori massage is called *mirimiri*) and eventually her pain went away.

"It was her grief, rage, sadness, and other huge emotions that got stuck in her body," Barrett says. "She had to stay strong for her children and couldn't process all her emotions, so this was the result."

> *"Grief, rage, sadness, and other huge emotions ... got stuck in her body."*

Barrett's client experienced one form of chronic pain, primarily driven by emotions, but there's a danger in thinking that women's pain has primarily to do with feelings. It touches on the widespread bias that women's pain is "all in their heads," that emotions and psychology are mostly to blame for their condition.

This is true for some women (and men), but doctors, the rest of the medical community, and society haven't caught up to the science, leading to dramatic disparities in how women's chronic pain is experienced, diagnosed, and treated.

141

In short, it sucks to be a woman in chronic pain because chances are you will be dissed, dismissed, and gaslit.

WHY ME?

This just in: I am not a woman.

Although I have chronic pain, I'm not ideally qualified to talk about how it feels to females. So, when I took up the topic of women and chronic pain, I turned to my wife (see Pain Profile: Was Her Pain Dismissed?), who also suffers from chronic pain, for insight.

I've also listened to and read about scores of women in pain — in interviews like the one with Barrett, in dozens of online support groups, in webinars on pain, in internet posts on Facebook and Reddit, and in articles in news, health, and lifestyle publications.

I was surprised, but not shocked, to learn that about seven in 10 people in chronic pain are female — at least that is what's widely reported. I see this in online support groups, including those hosted by the U.S. Pain Foundation and Chronic Pain Anonymous (see Sources of Solace), which are overwhelmingly attended by women.

A more authoritative stat comes from a study of Americans in pain in 2023, provided by the National Center for Health Statistics, that found women were more likely to have chronic pain (25.4%) than men (23.2%).

The chance of experiencing chronic pain conditions — such as fibromyalgia, migraines, chronic pelvic pain, autoimmune disorders, and rheumatoid arthritis, as well as conditions that affect females like endometriosis and menstrual pain — is greater for women than men. That's according to Kathy Sapp, Chief Operating Officer of the American Chronic Pain Association (see Sources of Solace), in a presentation during a webinar on "Women and Pain" I attended.

Sapp said:

> *Studies suggest that women report pain more frequently and often at higher intensity levels. [W]omen may receive less aggressive treatment for their pain compared to men. For example, women are less likely to be prescribed opioid painkillers or referred to pain specialists, and more likely to have their pain attributed to emotional or mental health issues.*

WOMEN EXPERIENCE CHRONIC PAIN DIFFERENTLY

The idea that women and men have different experiences of chronic pain is backed by other research, which has found:

- Women feel more chronic pain over their lifetimes than men

- They report more widespread pain in body parts

- Women are 10% less likely to have a recorded pain score on a scale of 0 (for no pain) to 10 (for the worst pain imaginable)

- Females ages 18 through 64 have a higher prevalence of multiple chronic conditions — called comorbidities — than men

"Women are less likely to get pain drugs."

- Women are less likely to get pain drugs (regardless of the gender of nurses or doctors) and they can experience profound stigma (see chapter 33).

In addition, women report more-intense pain and lower pain thresholds compared to males. (Those who've given birth may beg to differ with the latter.)

According to an article in *The Hill*:

> *Give someone an electric shock; bind a tourniquet tighter and tighter around their leg; submerge their hand in icy water; prick them with a pin: Researchers have done it all, and they've found — across years and hundreds of studies — that the same stimuli provoke greater pain responses in women.*

Despite that, the perception persists among many physicians that women can handle more pain than men. Women have reported receiving Tylenol after wisdom teeth removal, while men get opioids. Barrett said the same is true for cesarean sections and vasectomies.

The prevailing attitude among many is that pain is just part of being female and "being a woman is hard," a common refrain.

These sorts of differences disproportionately affect women of color, says an article on the website HealthyWomen:

> *People of color may be more likely to experience pain and to underreport their symptoms. ... To make matters worse, appropriate treatments may not be as available in communities of color. Healthcare providers continue to be misinformed*

about racial differences in the experience of pain, and implicit bias affects the management of pain. … Inadequate research into pain among women and people of color compounds the lack of understanding and resulting stigma.

Sapp also said there is bias in pain treatment of males and females:

Women often experience delays in receiving appropriate diagnoses for pain-related conditions. Their pain is sometimes dismissed or attributed to psychological factors, such as anxiety or depression, rather than being investigated thoroughly.

THE ROOT OF DIFFERENCES

Why do differences in the experience of pain between males and females occur? No one is exactly sure. It could have to do with hormones, genetics, and psychosocial factors such as trauma or stress. Pain and emotions are intimately related (see chapter 26).

The idea that women are mostly in pain because of psychological reasons, though, is a long-held myth that's used to dismiss them. That assumption is mistaken, according to landmark research conducted by the University of Arizona Health Services and published in the journal *BRAIN*.

Previously, everyone assumed that all humans feel pain in the same way. Not true, according to researchers at UA. They concluded that there are biological differences in the pain receptors of females and males. The breakthrough: the scientifically validated finding that there is a physical reason women and men experience pain differently. The lesson for doctors is that they might need to treat pain in an alternative way for women, possibly developing drugs specifically for females.

In other research at the University of California San Diego School of Medicine, scientists discovered that there are varied biological systems women and men use to relieve pain. Males battle pain by unleashing "endogenous opioids, the body's natural painkillers, [while] women rely instead on non-opioid based pathways."

Researchers speculated that this may mean that females are less likely to find relief from prescription opioids like morphine and fentanyl (see chapter 18). They may also be more likely to become addicted to those drugs because they can't find relief from standard doses.

Said Fadel Zeidan, PhD, professor of anesthesiology and Endowed Professor in Empathy and Compassion Research at UC San Diego Sanford Institute for Empathy and Compassion:

Dependence develops because people start taking more opioids when their original dosage stops working. … That may be one reason that females are more likely to become addicted to opioids is that they're biologically less responsive to them and need to take more to experience any pain relief.

WOMEN FACE SPECIAL BURDENS

Sapp touched on another special issue women in pain face — they are often wives, partners, or mothers who can't afford to take time to heal because of family responsibilities, which still predominantly fall on females. Whether due to nature or nurture, women tend to put everyone else's needs ahead of their own.

> *"Women tend to put everyone else's needs ahead of their own."*

Added Sapp:

> *Women with chronic pain are more likely to suffer from comorbid mental health conditions, including depression and anxiety. This creates a cycle where untreated mental health issues exacerbate pain, and chronic pain worsens mental health. The chronic nature of pain can lead to isolation, as women may withdraw from social activities, work, and relationships due to the physical and emotional toll of their condition*

This isolation and withdrawal have economic consequences — to women and the world. For example, a study of more than 17,000 women age 15 to 44 with endometriosis showed that more than two-thirds missed school or work due to their condition.

WOMEN IN PAIN AREN'T TAKEN SERIOUSLY

Doctors and others dismissing women's pain has been true for centuries, but you'd think that modern medicine would be more enlightened. Wrong. Bias endures even today.

An article on the website HealthyWomen explains:

> *There is the perception of the big, strong male who says he's in pain being taken more seriously by healthcare professionals and therefore acted upon [rather] than the weak little woman in the corner who is complaining about pain, and she's just had major surgery as well. She's often thought of as weak and not being able to tolerate pain or overstating her pain level.*

"Women fear being told pain is 'all in your head.'"

Women fear being told pain is "all in your head," but taken literally, it's true (see chapter 15). The brain processes pain and decides how bad it is. Unfortunately, the idea is weaponized against females to say their problems are psychological and emotional, rather than physical, making the conditions seem less serious.

Bias against women in pain care discourages them from seeking the treatments they need. According to a 2019 survey by HeathyWomen of 1,004 women who experienced persistent or recurring pain for more than three months:

- 90% received a diagnosis, with the most common ones including arthritis, migraine, fibromyalgia, autoimmune diseases, and pain from surgery and spinal disc issues

- 48% used opioids for pain relief

- 36% of respondents thought their healthcare provider did not take their pain seriously

- 62% of women sometimes felt hopeless and/or helpless about their pain

- 95% reported their pain affected their chance of living a full and active life

- 38% of respondents said they don't get enough information about pain.

Women face a lot of work to be taken seriously by healthcare providers, says a study documented in the journal *Social Science & Medicine*. When going to the doctor, they are often met with "skepticism and lack of comprehension, feeling rejected, ignored, and being belittled, blamed for their condition and assigned psychological explanation[s]."

Further, the research found females had to exert themselves to:

> *Attract the doctor's medical attention ... and were anxious to [not] be considered as whiners or complainers. ... Their efforts reflect a subtle balance not to appear too strong or too weak, too healthy or too sick, or too smart or too disarranged.*

HEALTHCARE BIAS AGAINST WOMEN

In the webinar I attended about "Women and Pain," Cynthia Toussaint talked about how doctors have told her in response to her complaints of pain, "Why don't you just shoot yourself in the head?"

Because of these kinds of shocking insults and attitudes, she founded the non-profit For Grace and its "Women In Pain Project," which advocates for women like her. Toussaint observed during the webinar:

> *Doctors see men as breadwinners and therefore more important. Women's psyches are so profoundly stained by gaslighting. We experience more mental health issues — anxiety and depression — as a result of this that we start questioning our own experience. As a result of gaslighting, we feel guilty as being overcomplainers; we stop going to doctors.*

GLIMMER OF HOPE

The pain situation for women is not hopeless. More research is being done on the pain females feel and their treatment by the healthcare community. Toussaint pointed out that in 2023, 55% of medical students were women. While women make up only 38% of today's physician workforce, their numbers have increased 26% from 2004 to 2022. Some research indicates women are just better doctors.

And women and their pain are getting more attention worldwide. For example, the International Association for the Study of Pain (IASP), the poobahs of pain research, named 2024 as the Global Year About Sex and Gender Disparities in Pain. This brought attention to equity issues in pain research, which often doesn't take into account gender.

My limitations as a man aside, it's clear to me that women like my wife are treated differently by doctors than I am. My confession: Call it white male privilege but I have never had my pain dismissed and I have comparatively little problem getting the medicine I need. I'm sorry that she, my daughters, grand-daughters, and other females face such barriers to equal healthcare.

It's a disgrace. It's disgusting. It stinks.

Maybe books like this will affect attitudes about the stark difference between how women and men experience pain and its treatment. I hope so.

I'll leave the last word to fitness coach Jana Barrett:

> *If you are a woman in pain, don't be afraid to speak up. I recommend that women get loud, assertive, and angry about having their pain dismissed or belittled.*

Pain Points

"Because I deal with fibromyalgia but to society 'look' healthy, it's been hard navigating my limits. ... Disability keeps denying me my right, but I also have the drive to do more. Physically I can't; mentally I can." —Blackintrovert

"I rarely had [my pain] taken seriously and had it most of my adult life. I think the gaslighting is true for people over 70 too. Men and women in my family have complained of pain and had serious terminal diagnoses overlooked because doctors have attributed their pain to ... aging." —Kay Flanagan

"Unfortunately for me. I had double jeopardy as a Black woman. When I needed surgery, the chief consultant was humble enough to admit his errors once he saw my pelvis. He used my success at work as an excuse to underestimate the impact of the symptoms. He was kind and apologetic and would have been horrified if accused of gender or racial bias. That was over fifty years ago and not much seems to have changed." —Verbieann Hardy

"Women should be respected and given more care. Women [are] in all forms of God — a mother, sister, wife, and so on. I strongly feel if we respect our Mother, then we'll respect any women in the world. Equality to all in all aspects." —Prem Sagar Sunchu

"As a chronic pain sufferer who is constantly ignored and belittled, ... I can attest to so much of this. From spine injury — solution 'stretch more' — to massive internal surgery while my husband had a minor knee repair. Ibuprofen for me, unlimited opioids for him. Surgeries within weeks of each other. Nothing is fair in pain for women." —Tabitha Warren

Pain Points are comments on this essay as it appeared originally on Medium.com. They are solely the opinions of the commentators and do not necessarily reflect the views of the book author or publisher.

20

Man Up

How males like me express and repress hurt

I screamed to the nurses, "Stop!"

They didn't.

Earlier in the day, at age 27, I'd had my first hip replacement (see chapter 11). To prevent bed sores, the nurses caring for me that evening decided to roll me onto my right side, opposite the hip that had been replaced.

Two of them got behind me and pushed. As I was rolled, I felt a stabbing, searing pain in the just-operated-upon left hip and running up my back and down my leg.

Although that roll likely took just a few seconds, it felt like forever.

And it hurt like hell.

My memory is of a frenzy of panic as the pain hit. What made it worse was my lack of control over my body, the feeling of helplessness as the nurses did their job. I was like a piece of meat at their mercy. I was truly terrified.

"I failed to follow the rules on my man card."

Afterward, I also felt deeply embarrassed.

By panicking, I failed to follow the rules on my man card. Like many males, I'd been raised to deal with pain stoically, without complaining or emotion. I had been conditioned to "man up," "rub dirt on it," and "get back in the game."

Most of all, I was told that boys don't cry.

How Men Can Deal With Pain

Based on my personal experience as a pain sufferer, here are some tips about how to deal with being a man in pain:

Learn to talk about pain
The strong, silent type is a male cliché. You may be reluctant to talk about your pain with a family member, a friend, or a counselor. But expressing pain and the emotions it brings is one of the best drug-free ways to lessen it. And learning the language of pain is particularly important when interacting with physicians, nurses, and other healthcare providers.

Take pain on as a project
Many men love projects and there is an enormous amount to learn about chronic pain if you look for it. I've taken it on as a personal project with the aim of creating this book about it. Even if you aren't writing about pain, learn about the science of pain, the ways it works within your body, and the biopsychosocial factors (see chapter 26) that can make it easier to live with.

Share the burden
One of the hardest things I've had to learn is how to share the burden of my pain with others, particularly my pushy wife (see chapter 2). Men are reluctant to ask for assistance (you know the pre-GPS cliché

I admit, though: That night I wept.

It was the worst pain I'd ever felt in a lifetime of chronic pain due to the genetic disease I inherited from my mother. The hip replacement that day was just the first of eight joint replacements I've had over the years.

My experience back then and throughout decades of chronic pain is an example of the complex relationship men have with hurt.

While women may be dissed, dismissed, and gaslit (see chapter 19) when it comes to chronic pain, men are taken more seriously by healthcare providers.

Yet our reluctance to admit we are in pain leads to unnecessary suffering and potentially more damaging disease.

HANDLING PAIN DIFFERENTLY

There's ample evidence that men and women handle pain differently.

On the one hand, research shows that over his lifetime the average man feels less pain than the average woman, partially because females live longer. On the other, how we males report pain may be just plain bulls***t.

The National Center for Health Statistics says:

> *The percentage of adults who had chronic pain and high impact chronic pain (pain that interferes with daily life) in the past three months was higher in women than men.*

Men were about two percentage points less likely to experience chronic pain, at 23.2%, than women, at 25.4%.

Other studies show a greater gender gap. About

one-third of men have chronic pain as compared to just under half of women.

According to research reported in *Time*, which studied pain reactions among 161,000 patients for 47 different disorders:

> [O]verall, women were more likely to indicate higher pain levels than men, said the [late] lead author Dr. Atul Butte, chief of systems medicine in the department of pediatrics at Stanford University School of Medicine. And that was true across almost all of the different diseases. 'That was the most surprising finding,' [Dr.] Butte says. 'We completely wouldn't have expected such a difference across almost all disorders, where women were reporting a whole pain point higher on the 0-to-10 scale than men.'

The stats aren't a value judgment about men and women. Pain strikes us all. And women can always talk about the trials of childbirth.

Given the differences in experience between men and women, the big question becomes *Why?* Here are some leading theories:

BIOLOGY

The idea that men and women experience pain differently tended to be dismissed in the past. After all, aren't all humans essentially the same? No. Not at all.

More recently, researchers found that chronic pain expresses itself differently in males and females based on biology. Boys and girls appear to have essentially the same pain reactions until puberty, when hormones enter the picture. Research shows, for example, that women's pain fluctuates based on where they are in their cycles.

about men never asking for directions). But keeping your needs to yourself results only in frustration. Learn to ask for help. There are people around you who love you and want to help. Maintain an attitude of gratitude and accept it graciously.

There's also some thought that testosterone is a natural painkiller, as opposed to estrogen. A study reported by *Pain Pathways* found:

> *Research in this area yields fascinating results. For example, male experimental animals injected with estrogen, a female hormone, appear to have a lower tolerance for pain — the addition of estrogen appears to lower the pain threshold. Similarly, the presence of testosterone, a male hormone, appears to elevate tolerance for pain in female mice: the animals are simply able to withstand pain better.*

Recently, scientists at the University of California San Diego School of Medicine discovered that men and women vary when it comes to pain. When hurt, they each use distinct biological systems.

Reported *Psychology Today*:

> *This may help explain why women seem more likely ... to experience chronic pain and tend to experience less pain relief from treatment with the most prescribed pain medications — opioids.*

The research results suggested that:

> *Men rely on endogenous opioids to reduce pain [while] women rely on non-opioid mechanisms to reduce pain. Endogenous opioids such as endorphins are the body's natural painkillers. These naturally occurring substances act similarly to prescription opioids like morphine, oxycodone, and hydrocodone, binding to opioid receptors in the brain to reduce the perception of pain. In contrast, pain relief for women appears to utilize alternative, non-opioid pathways, suggesting that women make less use of the body's internal opioids for pain relief.*

CONDITIONING

My experience as a man in pain is common. We males tend to be taught to shake off hurt and press on without complaining. It's possible that psychological conditioning from childhood makes males more resistant to pain or less likely to acknowledge it.

Many men see enduring pain silently as masculine. They are more likely to dismiss their pain as no problem. In my experience, a certain amount of hurt can also be invigorating, the old "no pain, no gain" theory of exercise.

Men may simply be less likely to talk about pain than women. I see this in Zoom chronic pain support groups I attend run by the U.S. Pain Foundation (see Sources of Solace). I am usually the only man among a group of a dozen or so women. I participate and talk about my pain, but sparingly, with the majority of the time going to others. It's a small, self-selected sampling, of course, but I've witnessed this gender gap consistently.

"I've witnessed this gender gap consistently."

The idea of enduring pain stoically is deeply ingrained in my male psyche. I have made a hobby of writing about chronic pain and the emotions that accompany it, but I admit I suffer from something of a psychological roadblock when it comes to admitting weakness.

Men are conditioned to see themselves in competition with others, particularly other males. Not admitting that they hurt might be some men's version of proving they are better, bigger, and stronger than the other guy. Consider the acclaim pro athletes get when they "give their bodies for the game" and "leave it all on the field."

It could be a way for men to feel better about themselves is by winning some kind of weird pain game: I'm tougher because I feel less pain than you (or I don't tell about my pain). This might also explain the well-known tendency among men to avoid doctors.

Given my disability due to genetic disease, I've come to rely on my wife for caregiving (see chapter 24), something I am extremely grateful for. But a part of me rebels at having to depend on another person; it's not in accord with how I think of myself as an independent, in-control man. I work hard at being able to accept help.

Like many men, overcoming my conditioning to be a strong, silent type is a barrier to my getting the help I need with my pain.

MISREPORTING

Researchers are handcuffed when it comes to studying chronic pain.

It can't be captured under a microscope or tested through blood or urine. An MRI or CT scan might show damage to the body, but doctors can't measure how that translates into pain. More technologically advanced fMRIs can show how parts of the brain activate when a person experiences pain, but, again, that can't be closely correlated with the patient's actual experience, and it's far too expensive and unwieldy to be used as a diagnostic tool.

Only recently have researchers discovered possible biomarkers for pain (see chapter 35).

The best tool physicians have to assess pain is to ask people what they feel. This tends to take the form of requesting that patients give a number between 0 and 10, with 0 being no pain and 10 being the worst pain imaginable. I've written about the problems with this pain scale in chapter 21, but when it comes to men, the issue may be that males misreport or downplay their pain to appear tougher.

> *"Males [may] misreport or downplay their pain to appear tougher."*

Each month, I visit a pain clinic to get a prescription for my fentanyl patches. The physician assistant I see asks for a number to measure my pain. I usually say 7 or 8, but I know I'm playing a pain game. Others may as well. Not only is the pain scale unreliable, but it's vulnerable to misreporting.

So, the pain gap between men and women may be due to bad data. It could be that males, consciously or unconsciously, consistently underplay their amount of pain.

FEELINGS OF FAILURE, SHAME, AND PURPOSELESSNESS

To me, and I'll wager to many other men like me, chronic pain feels like a personal failure in life.

This is backed up by Keith Orsini, quoted in *Pain Pathways*, who has complex regional pain syndrome (CRPS) and has worked with others with the disease:

> *Having talked to tens of thousands of CRPS patients over the last twenty years of both sexes, I see both sides. … We men haven't learned … to communicate our feelings … especially our feelings of failure. … Most men feel getting a chronic illness and ending up disabled … is a sign of failure when we can no longer provide for our families.*

The effects chronic pain can have on careers is crushing (see chapter 4). I was forced from mine at age 53 due to my disability. I wrestled with feeling ashamed that I couldn't make a good salary, instead relying on Social Security Disability Insurance to get by. I had so much of my identity wrapped up in my work as a writer, editor, and marketer that I became depressed and anxious (even more than usual) when it all went away. Adjusting took a full decade or so.

In general, we men define ourselves by what we can do. (Again, in general, there are always many exceptions.) We look at ourselves in terms of being useful and having a purpose.

Living in chronic pain can wipe away all that and leave us with feelings of purposelessness, inadequacy, and impotence. The physical changes it brings can harm our self-image (see chapter 9). For example, I used to be handy around the house, including remodeling a whole kitchen myself, but now I struggle with osteoarthritis in my legs, arms, and hands. I feel a profound sense of loss of the proficient person I used to be.

I deal with the fallout of my pain every day. Some of what I feel comes from my experience as a man. My pain is likely influenced by biology, but it also could be affected by my psychological conditioning, starting as a young boy. Even though I am a "words" guy, I struggle to report my pain in a complete, accurate way.

Why is this a problem? Men may be leaving relief on the table because they are reluctant to report pain. And small pain problems may become big ones without treatment. The results could be a more long-lasting and damaging disease.

But if we men really want to cope with chronic pain, we indeed need to "man up" and accept the help that's out there.

That's the truly manly thing to do.

Pain Points

"'Don't be a baby, suck it up' is one of the most common layman responses to a man saying he's in pain — and it frequently comes from women. Women tend to get acknowledged much more quickly." —Tim Consolazio

Pain Points are comments on this essay as it appeared originally on Medium.com. They are solely the opinions of the commentators and do not necessarily reflect the views of the book author or publisher.

21

Pain Scale Problems

*Rating chronic pain from
none to a ton is mostly useless*

The question comes monthly: "How's your pain?"

To get the drugs I need to manage my chronic pain, I visit a pain practice every 30 days. When my prescriber asks me about my pain each time, she isn't expecting a frank opinion such as, "It sucks."

No, she wants me to give a number between 0 (no pain) and 10 (the worst pain imaginable). (See illustration next page.)

That's when what I call "The Pain Game" starts.

Make no mistake: She genuinely cares how I feel and wants an honest answer. But, for me, the question is just too fraught.

> *"That's when what I call 'The Pain Game' starts."*

FUDGING THE SCORE

From my experience, patients get little guidance as to what a pain score is and how best to calculate it.

I wish my doctors had answered such questions as "What does the scale really measure?" "How do I choose a score?" and "Exactly how does my score affect my treatment?"

But they haven't. They just want me to give a number they can record in my chart and for my insurance company.

So, without clear guidance, intense calculations run through my mind: If I say a number that's too low, my prescriber may think that I'm fine (which I'm really not) and choose to restrict my prescription.

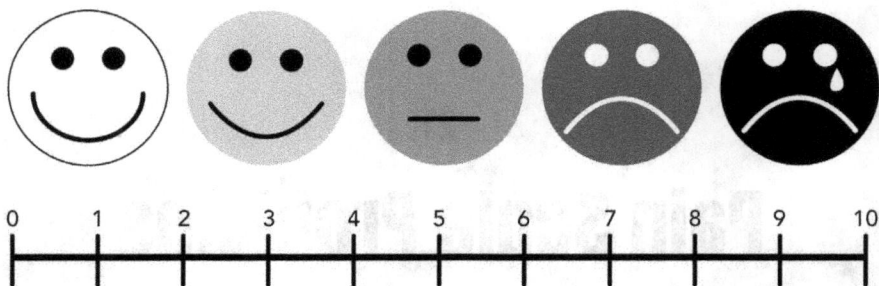

Illustration by Katie Schweiger

If I say a number too high — like that terrible 10 — then she might not take me seriously. If I were to name a number that large, I feel like I should be writhing on the floor crying uncontrollably because I hurt so much. If I report that, she may say to herself, "He's being so *dramatic*" (something chronic pain sufferers are accused of all the time).

Even answering 9 seems too high, not so much based on what I feel (sometimes my pain is a 9) but because it makes sense to leave some room if things go really wrong. It's like scoring figure skating at the Olympics; judges don't want to give early contestants a top score because someone later might do better.

So, I always say 7 or 8, judging that it will make my pain seem serious but not exaggerated. (Plus, I can certainly imagine pain worse than mine.)

Numbers from 3 to 6 just seem kind of a mid-score that says "medium" pain. The intensity of my pain and its effects on me are certainly not medium.

And I take 0 to 2 as meaning almost no pain at all, which happens only rarely for me.

POOR SCORES

Always reporting a 7 or 8 means my pain score doesn't change much from visit to visit, which is also true of my pain. It does vary from moment to moment within a day, from hour to hour, from day to day, from week to week, but measured over an entire month, it's always consistently poor.

And if she's asking me to rate my pain right at the exact moment I'm at the office, it's a pointless question. It may be the placebo effect, but I don't often feel my worst when in a physician's office. I mostly need treatment for all the other times when my pain is out of control.

When playing The Pain Game, I'm not being dishonest with my prescriber. I am, rather, guesstimating what will best communicate how I feel because I need my medication. I admit I am dependent on — but not addicted to — the opioid I use (see chapter 7). I am scared to death about what would happen if it were stopped and I had to go through violent withdrawal.

Risking that the pain practice — or, God forbid, a politician — might decide that my pain level is too low for my prescription is just too big a chance to take.

My prescriber knows that patients fudge their pain scores. She's sympathetic but wishes that everyone would be completely honest and correct.

The problem is that complete accuracy is impossible. There's no way to precisely numerically assess the sensations I or another patient feel. Pain is entirely too subjective.

"It's not like each of us has an internal pain-o-meter."

RATE YOUR PAIN

The rate-your-pain question puts too much onus on patients. It's not like each of us has an internal pain-o-meter that gives off a certain score.

The query is more likely to confound, confuse, and coerce people like me, rather than yield something scientifically accurate.

Aches, zaps, shocks, stabs, pins and needles, and other sensations vary in intensity, variety, impact, quality, quantity, and sheer ouch. They happen in our bodies, invisible to others, even if we have visible injuries that make other people wince for us.

We each have different pain thresholds. For example, research shows that, in general, men have higher pain tolerance than women (see chapter 20). Who really knows, though, whether pain among groups is at all comparable?

The truth is that my pain cannot be compared to your pain. Each is unique. My pain is mine alone.

For chronic sufferers like me, this means pain is terribly lonely (see chapter 16).

Being scientists and believing in the power of data, physicians, clinicians, and researchers continue their attempts to quantify pain. Most scales use the 0–10 model, like the one illustrated with happy faces ranging from a big grin to an agonized grimace (see above).

The limitations of these kinds of pain scales are many. According to an article from the Mayo Clinic Press:

> *Many pain scales focus on a person's pain level at the moment of the test and fail to address how pain affects people's daily life. For example, the scales often don't accurately assess these aspects of being in pain:*
>
> *Pain tolerance. Every individual's tolerance to pain is unique. It's shaped by biological and psychological factors — including genetics.*
>
> *Pain history. An account of previous or ongoing pain can inform how a person copes with pain and what treatments have worked in the past.*
>
> *Emotional state. Emotions can influence a person's pain scale ratings. In addition to pain, people often feel anxiety, anger, grief, stress and helplessness.*
>
> *Pain changes with activity. Pain may get better during certain activities and get worse with others. For example, a person with chronic back pain could feel worse after sitting at a desk all day and better after a yoga class.*
>
> *Pain fluctuations over time. Many pain assessments only reflect how much pain the person is feeling at the time of the test. It can increase or decrease with the time of day. Recent studies suggest it's more valuable to ask individuals to rate their average pain over a week or more.*

GARBAGE IN, GARBAGE OUT

"Doctors are given no better alternative."

The reason pain scales like the above persist is that doctors are given no better alternative. It's possible to see how pain affects the brain through fMRIs but results are far from cut-and-dried and expensive scans are impractical to do for most patients.

Researchers use assessments to do studies comparing pain across groups, but self-reported numbers are far from objective, unlike, say, blood pressure or cholesterol measurements. When it comes to aggregating data about pain, the old computer term GIGO applies — Garbage In, Garbage Out.

I can see one legitimate use of the 0-to-10 pain scale. It could measure how hurt changes over time for an individual. If, for example, a person's rating of acute pain reduces from 7 to 4 from one month to the next, it could mean healing.

Chronic pain, on the other hand, endures and often seems immune to getting better.

In her book *8 Steps to Conquer Chronic Pain: A Doctor's Guide to Lifelong Relief*, pain expert Andrea Furlan, MD, PhD, and professor of medicine at the University of Toronto (see Foreword), observes that the pain scale is useful, if not a bit problematic, for acute pain:

> *With chronic pain, measuring pain is even more challenging. The numbers do not make much sense when someone is always, constantly, in pain. For many, even when the pain is 4 out of 10, it is so tiring and annoying that it feels like 11 out of 10. Most of my patients would say that these questions do not make any sense to them, but unfortunately, we do not have a better method to assess pain intensity.*

But doctors and patients like me have no choice but to use a pain scale, which leads to playing pain games. It's inherently subjective, inaccurate, and ultimately pretty useless, but we settle for it because it's the best tool we have.

How's my pain? Still an 8.

Thanks for asking.

Pain Points

"[I] have had both chronic and traumatic pain (broken bones, arthritis, gut issues, car wrecks), and after the inane scale questions, I finally came up with the F Scale. The F Scale is based on how many "F***s!" I utter when the pain happens. A chronic ache that prevents me from exercising might be 2 small Fs, whereas an ax in the foot is definitely 10 Fs, especially the needle in the bottom of your foot to apply the numbing agent. Arthritis in wrists ranges from 3–8, depending on force and angle. Metabolism issues prevent me from taking pain meds usually, so unless I get surgery, I don't try to justify my F number. It's mostly for my own reference." —Auntiegrav

"I've always struggled with giving a number on the pain scale, especially when it feels like a 'good day.' The accumulative effect of living with some sort of pain for 20+ years takes its toll and can't be accurately captured on a 0 to 10 pain scale. There are just so many factors that go into how we're perceiving pain (and different types of pain) in any given day." —Caitlin Oliver

"When my uncle broke two vertebrae in his back, he always described his pain as a 10. I've read 'helpful' descriptions that said a 10 was that it hurt so bad he couldn't move

161

(which fit his condition) and others that said a 10 was that it hurt so bad the person was screaming and crying and writhing (that didn't fit his condition). What my uncle really meant was that it was the worst pain he had ever felt, including his many kidney stones. There has to be a better way." —Liza Jane

Pain Points are comments on this essay as it appeared originally on Medium.com. They are solely the opinions of the commentators and do not necessarily reflect the views of the book author or publisher.

Game Pain

A senior chronic pain sufferer turns to poetry to ease the hurt

Susan Hoffman feels tiny little yellow guys from a popular video game eat at her insides, causing her chronic pain.

The 64-year-old resident of Frisco, Texas, wrote a poem to describe the sensation:

Killer.

The mind, body, and soul.

Pain.

Never-ending, omnipresent,

Unrelenting,

Pain.

It chomps away the fabric that

helped my ability to avert, divert, or

re-arrange Its intensity.

A battle won and a battle lost:

Chomp,

by

> *"Never-ending, omnipresent, unrelenting, pain."*

Chomp.

The Pain has its own narcissistic grandeur,

demanding attention 24–7.

When my evasive tactics fail,

The Pain moves to a new level making all of my

distractions even more ineffective.

My internal pac-men of Pain.

Incessant.

Destructive.

Indestructible.

Bite by ever-present bite Pain wins,

It helps create the space for despair and hopelessness

to make their move,

It's the pervasive chomping, forever chomping,

destroying my fortresses one lethal bite

at

a

time.

Hoffman explains:

I attempt to write a type of poetry. It's mostly for me and/or my therapist. I wrote this one for myself out of a sense of desperation. Writing helps concretize the diffuse emotions that pain creates.

DECADES OF HURT

As a senior, Hoffman has dealt with chronic pain for four decades, since she injured her back at age 23. She recalls:

I was a home health aide. I was working with a man in the end stages of Parkinson's. I tried to transfer him to his wheelchair and didn't really have the strength or skill. I did eventually get him there, but the damage to my back was done.

Doctors fused herniated discs in her spine.

"I had the surgery and have never really been the same. My pain is achy, sharp, and burning, depending on my activity. If I've been too busy my pain ratchets way up. It impacts all aspects of my life."

She has had more than 10 surgeries over the years.

I have a nerve stimulator in my neck that is not as helpful as I had hoped. I had one in my lumbar but ended up with complex regional pain syndrome (CRPS). I've had multiple injections in both my lumbar spine and cervical spine. More than anything they gave very temporary relief, not as I had hoped, again. I go to psychotherapy and that helps relieve some of the depression that comes with intense chronic pain.

THE WORST THING ABOUT CHRONIC PAIN

Hoffman thinks the worst thing about chronic pain is:

The sense of feeling alone, trapped by the pain inside my body. With chronic pain, there's not only the physical component, but there's an emotional and spiritual factor. Chronic pain is almost a whole life experience, not one that I recommend to anyone. Some days, I feel like crawling in a hole and not coming out, ever.

"I feel stigmatized because of how unabated and insidious it is."

With regard to chronic pain, Hoffman has experienced a gamut of emotions.

She reports: "I grieve not being able to enjoy life as I'd like. I feel despair fairly regularly. When my pain increases, I feel like it's not worth this fight. Sometimes, I become furious about my pain. It's taken its toll on every aspect of my life and it just pisses me off."

"No one can take this pain away; it's invisible and not well-managed. I feel stigmatized because of how unabated and insidious it is. If I had cancer, as ironic as that is, it'd be more accepted," Hoffman adds.

Her advice to other pain sufferers is:

> *To not give up or give in to the pain, but that's easier said than done. Pain is exhausting and unremitting pain even more so. Talk to friends who understand that living in pain is not a thing for blame and shame but something that needs love and caring. Get outdoors when possible. There is a fair amount of scientific information that shows the benefit of being outside and joining with nature.*

And write, Hoffman concludes: "Write about what you are experiencing, what is happening now, and what it might be like to be pain-free. Fantasy is a good escape method."

22

Are You a Heartsink Patient?

Some pain sufferers deflate and defeat physicians,
but they are not the problem

Doctors have a name for patients they perceive as overly difficult, emotional, or obnoxious.

These folks are "heartsink" patients for how they make physicians' hearts drop when they are seen on the appointment schedule.

Heartsink patients may be "frequent flyers" who show up time after time with complex symptoms that are hard to pin down and treat.

Or they may let their feelings get the best of them and cry, complain, and seemingly crave attention.

Or they may be just seen as problematic (aka obnoxious — my word, not theirs).

And they may be people whose chronic pain can't be traced to a physical source or cured.

"A doctor coined ... 'heartsink patients' 40 years ago."

PHYSICIAN'S PROBLEM

A doctor coined the term "heartsink patients" about 40 years ago and it became popularized in an academic paper shortly after that, appearing periodically in medical literature since then.

I first came across the term when researching material for this book. Apparently pain patients, like those with hard-to-diagnose conditions, can easily fall into the heartsink category as they give into frustration and lash out.

To be clear, healthcare providers don't formally name problem people as heartsink patients. There is usually nothing in their files that refers to that. It's

How to Fight Against Heartsink

Though it's not a patient's responsibility to fix the feeling of dread among physicians, there are some things you can do if you suspect you have been labeled a heartsink patient:

Sketch out what you want to say to the doctor before an appointment
Come in with a plan. Write a note on paper, on your phone, or on the patient portal that explains precisely what's wrong. Resist generalities like "I don't feel well" and go for specifics like "I have a stabbing pain running down my right leg."

Seek providers with experience
Not to trash younger physicians and nurses, but the heartsink feeling tends to diminish as doctors and nurses get older and more seasoned. On the other hand, an experienced physician may be stuck in his or her ways. If one provider seems to be unfairly judging you, don't be afraid to switch.

Understand that doctors and nurses are human
The white coat can be off-putting but remember that these folks are just people with human attitudes and judgments. Give doctors and nurses some grace and relate to them as people.

more of a personal feeling, an internal judgment, a mental sigh.

You don't want to be caught in the trap of being a heartsink patient. There are ways to avoid that label (see sidebar).

The truth, though, is that the problem isn't really yours; it's your doctor's.

HOW HEARTSINK WAS BORN

"One of the earliest references to the 'heartsink patient' can be found in a 1986 issue of the *BMJ* [*British Medical Journal*], where Dr. C.G. Ellis argues that 'dysphoria' is the cause of heartsink," explains an article in *Insights+* from the *Medical Journal of Australia*. It continues:

> *Ellis points to many features of the heartsink patient … A file 'thicker than normal,' a multitude of complaints mixed in with various comorbid conditions, and one or more drug dependencies, despite all medications seemingly completely ineffective. The hallmark of dysphoria, Ellis tells us, is dissatisfaction and you are left trying to 'treat the untreatable.'*

A couple of years later, another UK–based doctor named Tom O'Dowd popularized the word "heartsink" in a five-year study of his most difficult patients. For O'Dowd, the word had the ring of truth to it, that feeling in the pit of his stomach when faced with certain problem people.

"Heartsink patients exasperate, defeat, and overwhelm their doctors by their behavior," O'Dowd wrote.

Reports an article in the *British Journal of General Practice*:

> *O'Dowd's paper described a study of 28 patients*

'considered to be heartsink' in his practice. Over six months, these patients were discussed by practice staff at ... lunchtime meetings. The stated function of these discussions was to share information, define problems, formulate management plans, and provide support for the [general practitioner] assigned to each patient. ... When the meetings ceased, only nine of the 28 heartsink patients had been discussed. O'Dowd determined that 'Inadvertently this has provided two comparison groups: one group who had a management plan and one whose care was unplanned and reactive.' Five years later, O'Dowd compared these two groups using outcome measures such as frequency of attendance and whether or not the patients were still 'considered to be heartsink.'

O'Dowd's study wasn't very scientific, but it did compare heartsink patients who got intervention versus those who did not. In general, the former group received improved care, resulting in fewer doctor visits, and fewer being called difficult.

The study showed heartsink can be eased if doctors and staff put in the work.

WHO'S THE PROBLEM, REALLY?

Like terms such as "hangry" (hungry and angry) or "crowdsourcing" (getting a group of people to contribute cash to a project), "heartsink" conjured a mental image most everyone can relate to. It's a sort of nausea we get when going into an unpleasant situation, a feeling of dread.

It captured a real phenomenon among physicians and staff, seeing some patients as more challenging than others, whether due to personality or complexity of their problems. It resonated with healthcare workers as truly capturing what they often feel.

Build a relationship
You and your doctors have a professional relationship and it's good to respect boundaries. Still, you can build a rapport with them that goes beyond the mere exchange of information. The more they can see you as an individual — not a disease or injury — the better. Communication is key. So is trust-building.

Don't lash out
As hard as it can be when you are sick and frustrated, keep your emotions in check. Convey the seriousness of your situation but avoid letting them get the best of you.

Be persistent but polite
In my book research, I've heard scores of stories about people being ignored or misdiagnosed for years, sometimes decades. If you know something is wrong, stand up for yourself.

At the same time, though, always be courteous. Your goal is to get help, not to piss off providers.

Over time, though, critics derided the term as discriminatory, dismissive, and divisive.

The problem? Referring to heartsink patients puts them in an unfair box. "It is the doctor's heart that sinks, but it is the patient who receives the label," summarizes a paper in the *British Journal of General Practice*.

In other words: It's not necessarily that the patient is objectively problematic; the sinking feeling is a weakness of physicians. It says more about the doctors than it does the patients. Still, the patient bears the burden of the judgment, and that can bring negative consequences.

CONSEQUENCES FOR PATIENTS

Among the negative outcomes, reports a 2024 article in the *BMJ*:

> *The clinician can become defensive and adopt social limiting strategies, ignoring other cues, curtailing discussion, and cutting consultations short. … These approaches can result in a patient's passive acceptance of treatment, inappropriate interventions, and worse outcomes for the patient. There's a risk of care bouncing between clinicians, the central problem remaining unresolved, inappropriate referrals, clinical errors, increased overall workload, and overuse of appointments.*

There is good news, though, states the *BMJ*:

> *Training and wider workplace conditions can influence doctors' experience of the 'heartsink' feeling. Studies have found that experienced GPs tend to have fewer heartsink consultations and might even view these patients as a challenge and an opportunity to look for a successful outcome. Doctors with longer working hours and a higher number of patients with psychosocial or substance misuse problems were more likely to report feeling frustrated with patients. Heartsink is also reported more in doctors with less training in communication skills and fewer postgraduate qualifications. Better training and less stressful working environments therefore seem to have a protective effect against doctors' feelings of frustration.*

In other words, that sinking sensation is a signal to doctors that they may be doing something wrong in relating to patients. And it can be turned around.

"The heartsink feeling can be minimized and can even become a glorious 'heartrise' feeling when doctors unlock a problem or create a way forward with their patients," reports the *BMJ*.

Rather than looking down on patients and delivering inferior care, physicians should take it as a chance for professional growth and improving their practice.

But not all do.

A PATIENT SPEAKS OUT

Dawn Sharples suffers from myalgic encephalomyelitis/chronic fatigue syndrome (ME/CFS), which has led to many doctor and hospital visits. She fears physicians think of her as a heartsink patient, but she wants the public to know there is another side to the story.

> *"It is a rather derogatory term for patients who are seen as a pain in the backside."*

She writes in *The Mighty*:

> *If you aren't familiar with the phrase 'heartsink patient,' it's a rather derogatory term for patients who are seen as a pain in the backside and you get that 'heartsink' feeling when they enter the office. … These patients are never 'happy,' never get better, just keep coming back! But before you feel sorry for those overworked GPs and their difficult workload, listen to the other side of the desk.*

Sharples has been called attention seeking and overly anxious when she uses healthcare. She argues that she doesn't like hospitals or doctors. She's not bored or lonely. She continues:

> *The only reason I would consider going to the hospital is if I believe my life is in danger. Four times the hospital sent me home on the verge of heart failure, twice they sent me home with acute pancreatitis (it will kill you if not treated), four times they sent me home saying it was impossible for my condition to have progressed the way I was claiming (which it had and it was potentially fatal). … Every time I was treated like I was a time waster, attention seeker, told that I needed to get serious psychiatric help or that I didn't love my kids and wanted to get away from them. That is abuse, it is gaslighting, belittling behavior dealt out by someone in complete control of your life.*

Sharples makes clear that she doesn't believe all doctors and nurses behave like that but notes that even the most well-intentioned ones can "slip into institutional abuse. People who label patients as 'heartsink' or 'frequent flyers' … don't see them as fellow humans anymore, just a problem to be passed on as soon as possible."

She fears being labeled "overanxious," which can become a self-fulfilling prophecy. "You know once you panic, or start to cry, you might lose all respect from the doctor and become a problem no one wants," Sharples concludes. "An overanxious, crying, hysterical woman with a complicated medical history."

Don't get heartsick at the thought of doctors and nurses seeing you as a heartsink patient.

Treat providers as human beings and they'll likely do the same for you.

Pain Points

"I just went through an experience where I was sent home three times from one ER to finally be admitted to gall bladder surgery the 4th time at a different hospital at the recommendation of my endo surgeon. ... Prior to this [the first hospital] always treated me with respect but as I kept returning for a problem they didn't see as urgent, I saw how the nurses and staff changed their tune. I was accused of drug seeking, then anxiety, even though my pelvic [physical therapist] insisted I go back due to extremely high blood pressure. ... Finally, the last ER admitted me for accelerated ... hypertension that can lead to threat to life or body. It was the pain that was the emergency."
—Tracey Chester

"It's extremely difficult to remain calm at times when doctors don't believe you or [seem to] treat you with disdain. I do believe it comes from the doctor's unease with their own lack of ability to help or feeling as if their expertise is being challenged. When you're suffering as deeply as people with [problems like] ME/CFS often are, regulating emotions is beyond difficult. Imagine how hard it is for an average person to regulate their emotions when they've missed just one night of sleep. Now multiply that by about one thousand." —Kelley George

"The whole system sets physicians up to feel like this, and patients to be frustrated. Doctors don't have time to form a holistic picture of a patient; they have time only to order diagnostic blood tests and throw a medication at the most glaring symptom. If the patient asks to be treated as a full human being with interacting body systems and has an idea about how their symptoms are related, they are dismissed, because [mainstream] medicine by its nature is compartmentalized. It's frustrating and maddening for doctors and patients alike." —Dana Mayer

"Although you may perceive your doctor as brushing you off, they are following the algorithm for differential diagnosis that is ingrained in us from the beginning of medical school; get this lab test, assess this physical exam, order this imaging." —Kegan Cox

"I'm guessing the term 'heartsink patient' is synonymous with a female patient who expects to be treated and won't accept her obviously physical ailments being labeled 'psychosomatic' because doctors haven't bothered to study female physiology for the last 3,000 years." —Screen name withheld by request

Pain Points are comments on this essay as it appeared originally on Medium.com. They are solely the opinions of the commentators and do not necessarily reflect the views of the book author or publisher.

23

Weather or Not

Does climate cause pain?

Debby kicked my ass.

She caused my whole body to ache. She stabbed me in the right back of my neck and gave me a stress headache at the front of my skull. She made my right leg throb and vibrate. She attacked my lower back with spasms above the waistline. She even inflamed the knuckles of both my hands. All the pain nauseated me.

Debby was a hurricane, wind, and water that drenched the East Coast in 2024. It made landfall as a Category 1 in Florida, then traveled as a tropical storm through Georgia, the Carolinas, and up to the Northeast, including the Philadelphia area, where I live. Here, she brought steel-gray skies, up to 10 inches of steady rain over a couple of days, and a tornado that touched down in nearby Delaware.

It also made the chronic pain I deal with every day a lot worse.

Some days are worse than others. Chronic pain isn't a steady state. It changes by the moment, hour to hour, day to day, week to week. Before Debby, I'd had a run of not-as-bad days — until the clouds and showers came.

"I feel a storm acomin' in my bones."

Ask most chronic pain sufferers or their physicians and they'll say harsh weather worsens their hurt. When I chat with fellow chronic pain people on particularly grody days, they agree this happens all the time.

It's like what farmers have reported for generations, saying "I feel a storm acomin' in my bones."

WHAT EXPERTS SAY

Why? Is there a connection between climate and chronic pain, as anecdotal evidence — and my body — seems to show?

Cue the experts. Some confirm there is a link between bad weather and hurt, sort of. According to an article from the Cleveland Clinic:

> *Is there really a cause-and-effect relationship between weather and joint pain or is it just an age-old medical myth? For an answer, let's check with chiropractor Andrew Bang, a doctor of chiropractic at Cleveland Clinic. Judging by what Dr. Bang hears, the answer seems to be yes. 'I see it all the time in my office,' he says. 'People come in on bad weather days and they're like, 'I'm feeling it today. I'm really feeling it today.'*

The article cites a study of 13,000 people in the United Kingdom that found those with illnesses like arthritis hurt more when there was higher humidity, lower barometric pressure, and stronger winds. It continues:

> *But as is often the case, nothing is 100% when it comes to research. Other studies show just a casual or mild relationship between changing weather and achy joints.*

> *'So, is the belief about weather changes causing joint pain true?' asks Dr. Bang. 'Well, it doesn't happen to every person — but we know it happens to some. There's something there. We just haven't quite figured it out scientifically yet.'*

The Cleveland Clinic article also includes a theory of how bad weather brings more pain:

> *Decreasing pressure — which typically ushers in worsening weather — means air presses a little less on our bodies. That lack of compression allows tissues within your body to swell slightly, which can irritate your joints.*

> *The speed at which the pressure changes also makes a difference. A sudden drop in pressure as a storm blows into town creates more noticeable aches than a slow, gradual pressure decline.*

> *'So, if you have arthritis, the space in your joint is already reduced,' notes Dr. Bang. 'Add in an expansion of tissues because of the pressure change and you can see why people might hurt more.'*

HOW WEATHER IS LIKE CLOTHES

It's like the difference between a loose pair of shorts and spandex. In the latter case, the fabric is similar to high air pressure holding joints, ligaments, and muscles in place.

Other scientific studies generally back up the idea that weather can affect pain. One found that people who broke bones reported increased hurt with poor weather conditions a year later.

> *"It's like the difference between a loose pair of shorts and spandex."*

Another concluded:

> *Our study 'Cloudy with a Chance of Pain' analyzed daily data from 2,658 patients collected over a 15-month period. The analysis demonstrated significant yet modest relationships between pain and relative humidity, pressure, and wind speed.*

The arthritis website creakyjoints.org reports:

> *One study from Tufts University showed that with every 10 degrees drop in temperature, arthritis pain increased in the study participants. It also showed that low barometric pressure, low temperatures, and rain can increase pain. Studies in cadavers have showed that barometric pressure can affect pressure in the joints. In one cadaver study, low atmospheric pressure threw the ball of the hip joint off track by more than one-third.*

Creakyjoints goes on to say that multiple studies show that people tend to acclimate to where they live:

> *One study that looked at chronic pain sufferers in warm and cold areas — San Diego, Nashville, Boston, and Worcester, a Massachusetts city with much colder temperatures than Boston — found that two-thirds believed the weather worsened their pain. However, the perceived effect of weather on pain was not found to be related to the regional climate.*

So, climate may not worsen pain. The website says other studies show no difference in pain based on weather.

SAD TIMES

We know that pain affects depression (see chapter 10) and vice versa. Gray days can bring the blues and conditions such as seasonal affective disorder (SAD), boosting physical and emotional pain.

Even though the science is wishy-washy, we should trust all the chronic pain sufferers who say they hurt more when low pressure systems come through their communities.

I certainly do. Rainy days beat me up.

Good riddance, Debby.

Pain Points

"There are mornings I wake up in deep pain, and I know rain is on its way. It's as if my body carries a weather forecast of its own. Strange how pain becomes a kind of intuition." —Sahaj Bains

Pain Points are comments on this essay as it appeared originally on Medium.com. They are solely the opinions of the commentators and do not necessarily reflect the views of the book author or publisher.

24

Take Care

*My life with chronic pain is eased by my wife,
my caregiver, my love*

I hate to admit it — mostly because of my male pride — but I depend on my wife to get through the day.

She makes the meals that feed me. She washes the clothes I wear. She drives when we go out and about. She's my caregiver.

None of this is because I believe in any of that "trad wife" stuff you see on social media. It is not her purpose to serve me. MeK is a fully formed, mature adult who has her own dreams, opinions, and values.

Now retired due to burnout, she had a career as a freelance writer for a variety of publications, including *National Geographic Traveler*, for four decades. She takes care of herself and hits the YMCA most weekdays, meaning she can probably outmuscle me. She reared three daughters,

> *"It is not my pride that gives her life meaning."*

who now have given us two granddaughters. Although we worked together on parenting, I give her all the credit for the caring, independent, and accomplished people they've become.

Overall, I am so proud of her, but it is not my pride that gives her life meaning. She is so much more than just a "wife."

'TIL DEATH DO US PART

It turns out that MeK is among about 5.7 million spousal or partner caregivers in the US, according to the Well Spouse Association (WSA), whose mission is to "provide resources to spousal caregivers to help them manage their journeys a little more easily."

179

That's out of 53 million or so American adults who tend to a spouse, elderly parent, or special-needs child, a leap upward from 43.5 million in 2015. Women make up 56% of caregivers versus 44% men.

MeK is one of those female caregivers. She is tethered to me because she truly loves me (and I truly love her) and she made a commitment to me when we married almost 40 years ago. Although she isn't a practicing Roman Catholic anymore, she was raised in an Irish-American household that took vows seriously.

Want to know the secret of a long marriage? Don't get divorced.

Hang in there despite the ups and downs of all human interactions. Nobody should stay in a terrifying, toxic, or traumatizing relationship, but marriage is cyclical. It's made up of days when you are deeply in "like," which is more important than love long-term, ones in which the relationship is merely *meh*, and others where you can't stand the other person. It ebbs and flows. Success is not eternal happiness, but rather the satisfaction of building a life together.

A LIFE FILLED WITH CHRONIC PAIN

If you saw me sitting in my La-Z-Boy, you'd think nothing was wrong with me. I look like a normal 60-something man. But when I stand up and try to walk, you'd see I am hunched forward and use a HurryCane to get around the house. Follow me into the world and you'd notice I use a wheelchair because I can't tread more than a hundred feet or so at a time.

Throughout all my health issues, my wife has been there, encouraging, supporting, and caring about me while also caring for me.

I feel major guilt, and a bit of shame, for all she does for me. I try to say "Thank you" whenever she helps me. If she didn't have to spend her time taking care of me, she might be out hiking (which she loves) or traveling to see friends. My disability keeps her mostly tied to me and our home.

Recently, I shared these feelings with her, and she replied that they go both ways:

I feel guilty when I inevitably feel tired or overwhelmed or taken for granted or some FOMO (fear of missing out) after hearing about your brother and his wife's travels to the Galapagos or seeing photos on social media of some friend of mine posted from a hike or adventure experience with their partners. For me, at least, part of not becoming bitter or burned out as your caregiver is to be able to acknowledge these natural and honest feelings without guilt or judgment.

Whether that's voicing them to you or to a friend or to one of my brothers, it helps me feel heard and seen. That doesn't change anything or mean I resent you, it just lets me know I don't have to be Mother Teresa.

I followed up by asking her whether she feels trapped: "I didn't sign up for this. But I love the life we've built together, our kids and grandkids, our daughter-in-law and sons-in-law, our friends, our dog, our home. I'm not going anywhere."

> *"I don't have to be Mother Teresa."*

The truth is MeK's a natural caregiver, sometimes to a fault. I don't say this in the sense often used to dismiss women, that they are just better nurturers than men and that somehow their emotional labor is worth less. Whether nature or nurture, MeK truly cares about others. She volunteers to help those in need at our church and delivers for Meals on Wheels, for example.

Since retiring in 2021 she's taken care of our oldest granddaughter while my youngest daughter and son-in-law build careers and make a living. Three generations live in the same 2,400-square-foot house in the Philadelphia suburbs along with our dog and their cat. It can be chaos sometimes, but MeK is the emotional and practical center that keeps the circus churning.

CAREGIVING CONSEQUENCES

On its website, the Well Spouse Association (WSA) points out some unique aspects of caring for a spouse or partner:

- Such caregiving "tends to be higher intensity than other types of caregiving. It is more medically intensive, and spouses or partners support more activities of daily living (ADLs) for care recipients."

- 49% of spousal caregivers have cared for more than three years; 29% have been caregivers for more than five years; 14% for more than 10 years.

- Two out of three spouse or partner caregivers provide care without any unpaid or paid help as compared to 29% for other types of caregivers.

- Often the "patient and the caregiver must give up paid employment (at the same time that expenses increase due to medical needs)."

- "Spouses are often excluded from federal, state, and local services and supports available to other caregivers."

The WSA goes on to say:

The transition to caregiver/patient roles often includes the loss of a singular intimate relationship and its companionship. Spousal caregiving impacts the decision to have children, the way children are raised, and where and how one lives and retires. There are few areas of life that are left untouched by the caregiver/patient role in these relationships.

> "*There are few areas of life that are left untouched by the caregiver/patient role in these relationships.*"

Another resource for caregivers is a Zoom support group offered by Pain Connection, a program of the U.S. Pain Foundation (see Sources of Solace). Sign up under Specialized Support Groups on its website.

OUR NEWFOUND INTIMACY

MeK and I are lucky. Our caregiving relationship started in earnest in our 50s, somewhat later in life, after our kids finished college and launched into the world. And what she does for me is fairly mild compared to those who may have a spouse or partner with breast cancer, Parkinson's, or dementia.

Although there is stress on our relationship, there have been no crises that have torn us apart. I hope that continues as we age, but I know my condition might grow worse or that she might not be able to care for me — or I for her — as the years go by (she fears getting Alzheimer's like her mother).

It's true that our intimacy has suffered from both my physical problems and her chronic pain due to an accident that burned her right forearm and hand (see Pain Profile: Was Her Pain Dismissed?). But in a way, our emotional intimacy has increased as we've gotten closer by spending so much time cooperating and collaborating to deal with my disability.

I confess: It's difficult to depend on someone else. MeK has seen me at my most helpless, hapless, and humbled. I have given her power over me, which is hard for a man. She pushes me around, in my wheelchair (see chapter 2). When riding in it, I am not really in charge of the direction we're going — and I like being in control.

Sometimes when we're out in the world with the wheelchair, we'll pass people with young children in strollers. I sometimes feel infantilized and embarrassed by riding around like a toddler. It's been hard to come to terms with my lot in life.

The bottom line, though: The complete trust I place in MeK is the most intimate part of our marriage. When I asked her about our relationship, she said:

> *It hasn't been easy, but we've grown closer over the years that you've been disabled. I've had to stay strong for you and, frankly, it's sometimes exhausting to do all that physical and emotional work. I get tired. But I hang in there because, as you've said, 'We're bonded by the barriers we've faced.' [See chapter 2.] I care about you, and you care about me.*

And I keep in mind our caregiving relationship is healthy for me.

According to a study of 163 couples in which one partner had rheumatoid arthritis, the patients who reported high "dyadic coping," (that is, "the process of coping that transpires between couples challenged by one partner's illness") had lower rates of "depression, anxiety, and stress, and higher relationship quality; whereas participants who reported higher negative dyadic coping reported higher depression, anxiety, and stress, and lower relationship quality." The well partners also said they have greater rates of relationship satisfaction when they and their hurt partners coped well together than those whose significant others did not.

In nonacademic words, the study showed that close, concerned, and cooperative relationships between partner patient and well caregiver make both parties happier and healthier.

24 PLACES IN 2024

My wife's present to me on Christmas 2023 was to visit "24 New Places in 2024." We spent the year going on day trips and overnights all over eastern Pennsylvania, Delaware, Maryland, and even down to D.C. (the National Museum of African-American History and Culture).

None were big, life-changing treks and we were limited to places that are accessible to my wheelchair. Some were as easy as walking around the downtown of historic towns (such as New Castle, Delaware; Harve de Grace, Maryland; and Lititz, Pennsylvania), visiting museums (such as the National Museum of Industrial History, Bethlehem, Pennsylvania, and the Mercer Museum, Doylestown, Pennsylvania); and touring gardens (such as Mt. Cuba Center, Hockessin, Delaware).

MeK has become expert at finding accessible places and planning itineraries that we can do together. She puts her experience as a travel writer to good use as we explore. And she stays in shape as she uses her 100 pounds to push her 180-pound husband in the wheelchair (hills are a challenge). I joke that people should "feel my wife's thighs."

Sometimes there are inaccessible hiking or walking trails at places we visit, ones that MeK would enjoy trekking if she didn't need to stay with me. I regret that she can't do everything she would like because of my handicap. She's said that she isn't missing anything; she prefers staying with me.

The point of 24 in '24 was not to have grand adventures like skydiving. It was simply to be together seeing new things, talking or listening to podcasts in the car, and finding cool places to eat (her latest find was a roadside pierogi shop).

Everyday life around the house can get tense, but every time we get away we remind ourselves we are best friends.

Simple pleasures. Together. Take care.

Outdueling Pain

*After a freak event, a master fencer comes
to terms with his new life*

March 8, 2009, was a long day for Jim Ferrone — one that would permanently change his life.

The 50-year-old resident of Flemington, New Jersey, was in "fantastic shape," he says. After taking several weeks recovering from elbow surgery, he was at his college weight, ate healthy foods, and didn't smoke or drink, not even caffeine.

As an A-rated epee fencer (the top skill rating) and coach, Ferrone spent that day organizing and competing in a tournament.

"I did okay, 10th place," he recalls.

He was so exhausted that when he got home about 5 p.m. he collapsed on his living room carpet. His dog, Shiloh, jumped on his chest and started licking his face, something the 9-pound Chihuahua/Italian greyhound mix had never done.

Ferrone remembers: "I turned my head sharply to the right to avoid him and felt a crunch in the back of my neck. After a heartbeat, my head exploded in pain."

"After a heartbeat, my head exploded in pain."

Ferrone struggled to get the dog off him and laid there for five minutes before going upstairs to get some Tylenol. When he tried to go back down, he found his left leg was weak, his balance shot.

"My wife had to help me down to the couch," he remembers. "We called our doctor to ask what we should do, and she said to go to the emergency room."

185

MEDICAL ODYSSEY

After a monthslong medical odyssey that involved several physicians, a misdiagnosis, a rehabilitation facility, and multiple spinal taps, CT scans, MRIs, and more, doctors finally said Ferrone had experienced a vertebral arterial dissection (VAD), resulting in a stroke.

"Turning my head sharply dissected the artery that feeds my brain stem," he reports. "Some doctors have told me this is impossible, or close to it. It just doesn't happen, but it happened to me."

Ferrone spent time in a hospital trying to recover. In the predawn hours one morning, a new roommate arrived. The large, 60-something patient was given some food and immediately started gagging — "loudly" — which irritated Ferrone.

Breakfast caused the same reaction and it went on all day until Ferrone was discharged late in the afternoon. He says:

> *It got me really agitated, and triggered hiccups. They lasted for two weeks. This might have been the worst part of the stroke; it was horrible, exhausting, painful, just awful. They finally went away with medication. To this day, I panic if I get a hiccup.*

About three months after the stroke, Ferrone began to feel pain throughout his left side, which has been chronic ever since:

> *There is a constant burning sensation and I no longer feel skin temperature correctly there. I interpret too hot or too cold feelings as pain. If you ran water on my left hand, I couldn't tell the difference between hot and cold, only that it was too much one way or the other, and that it hurt.*

Then, a new pain developed in his left foot.

> *Fast forward to 2021. I had put on weight, so I started going to the gym with my wife. After a month, I noticed a bad pain in my little toes. I stopped exercising, but the pain got worse and spread.*

Over the following year, he saw 17 different doctors, including four podiatrists, three neurologists, two pain management specialists, a rheumatologist, and an endocrinologist, "but nobody could figure out what was wrong."

ONGOING SAGA

Finally, Ferrone found a neurologist who concluded he had Wallenberg's lateral medullary syndrome.

Basically, when he worked out too hard (his doctors theorize), the damage from the stroke in the thalamus moved and now presses on a nerve that transmits pain signals to his feet.

He says the foot problem is his greatest challenge right now. He is in constant pain: "a 4 on the pain scale, but it will go higher at times." The pain is dull, can radiate to his ankle, and occasionally up his entire leg.

"It feels like I'm stepping on jagged rocks."

"When I walk, it feels like I'm stepping on jagged rocks," Ferrone says.

In addition, he suffers from random face stabs, which tend to happen under his right eye or around his nose or cheek on that side. Ferrone adds: "They are quick, but intense. Sometimes they will linger for a minute or so. I apply pressure to get a little relief until they pass. I also have constant head pain."

Ferrone has tried a variety of treatments for his chronic pain, including two spinal stimulators that eventually "did nothing," medication, physical therapy, acupuncture, and injections — all without significant results. "I have tried essentially everything at least once" he says, "and nothing touches the pain."

REACHING RELIEF

Ferrone has gotten the greatest relief from seeing a counselor who taught him breathing exercises and other ways of steering his thoughts away from the pain He observes:

> *Counseling isn't going to take away my pain, but it does help me to deal with it better. It might not be for everyone, but if you are truly willing to do it and find someone that you really connect well with, it can be an incredibly positive experience.*

Ferrone has also tried online support groups but has a warning for other pain sufferers.

> *Support groups can be extremely helpful and make you feel less alone. However, you also hear story after story about people at the lowest point in their lives. It can be too much. If you are in despair about others all the time, it becomes more difficult to help yourself.*

187

Ferrone was a training coordinator for a medical device manufacturer, but in 2025 he was abruptly let go because the company said it was a safety issue for him to use his cane on the factory floor, despite his doing that without incident for the previous four years. He wants to get across how difficult it is to get others to understand his chronic pain:

> *That might be my thesis statement with all this: It's exceedingly difficult to describe chronic pain, your pain, to someone who doesn't experience it. This includes doctors and even other sufferers. I have had to explain it to at least 30 different medical professionals. You kind of develop a script after a while.*

Ferrone thinks that the worst thing about having chronic pain is that it limits him permanently:

"You kind of develop a script after a while."

I can't go back to what I was. I can never coach fencing again. I can't play pickup basketball or football with my family. It stops me from doing things that I really enjoy.

DON'T GIVE UP

Still, through counseling and his own inherent "don't-give-up" attitude, Ferrone has come to terms with his pain: "I accept that I might be in pain for the rest of my life, while also not giving up hope that something will come along someday that will help."

Because of his experience, Ferrone devotes some of his free time to spreading stroke awareness. He says it's therapeutic to tell his story to others, especially if they might be helped by it.

"After my stroke, it was years before I really talked about it," he explains. "It took my friend Mitch Davis dying of a stroke for me to realize I had this information that could save a life, so I have been an advocate of stroke awareness since."

Ferrone's fencing club, Bucks County Academy of Fencing (BCAF), holds an annual event in memory of Davis.

> *We did a fundraiser the first year. I thought we might be able to raise a couple hundred bucks, but we wound up raising over $6,000 for the National Stroke Association [now merged with American Stroke Association]! It was quite an experience, and it feels good to turn a negative into a positive.*

Part III: Relieving Chronic Pain

"Although the world is full of suffering, it is full also of the overcoming of it."

— *Helen Keller*

"Behind every beautiful thing, there's been some kind of pain."

— *Bob Dylan*

"There is a saying in Tibetan, 'Tragedy should be utilized as a source of strength.' No matter what sort of difficulties, how painful experience is, if we lose our hope, that's our real disaster."

— *Dalai Lama*

Source: Wisdomquotes.com

25

Why Sufferers Hate Yoga

'Have you tried that yet?'
and other unwelcome questions

The Zoom support group I attended broke into knowing groans.

The 10 or so participants, including me, suffer from chronic pain. We all had heard the same suggestion from family members, friends, coworkers, healthcare providers, even strangers: "Have you tried yoga yet?"

The question is sincere and comes from a genuine desire to help those of us in pain. But it is almost always not what chronic pain sufferers care to hear. The sentiment from us generally is, "Down with downward dog."

"Down with downward dog."

If you know someone in chronic pain — say a family member, friend, or coworker — it's vital to understand that the questions you ask may be unhelpful, unwelcome, or even hurtful. Honestly, we sufferers don't want to be pestered by so-called solutions we've been asked about before. It's exhausting to keep saying, "Yeah, I tried that and it didn't help much."

It's damaging to be constantly on the hook to explain why we aren't getting better right away. And it's demoralizing to be thought of as "not trying hard enough."

CURING VERSUS COPING

It isn't that yoga is bad for us (see sidebar). Some sufferers swear by it as a positive way to reduce stress, increase mobility and flexibility, and distract the mind.

"Yoga can help people with arthritis, fibromyalgia, migraine, low back pain, and many other types of chronic pain conditions. … Practicing yoga also improved mood and psychosocial well-being," according to an article from Harvard Medical School.

Yoga for Pain: What the Science Says

I don't mean to trash yoga. It's the constant suggestions that we chronic pain sufferers try it or other supposed fixes that's the irritation.

That raises the question, though: Can yoga really help ease enduring hurt? Scientific studies have found a so-so improvement in reported pain from doing yoga—enough to give it a try if you are healthy and mobile enough. There are also other mental health benefits.

Here's how different conditions respond, according to the following public domain information from the National Center for Complementary and Integrative Health released in 2024:

Fibromyalgia
Recent systematic reviews and randomized clinical trials provide encouraging evidence that some mind and body practices such as yoga may help relieve some fibromyalgia symptoms.

Low Back Pain
For patients with chronic low-back pain, recent evidence-based clinical practice guidelines from the American College of Physicians gave a strong recommendation based on moderate-quality evidence that clinicians and patients should initially

Fair enough. So why do pain sufferers hate being asked the yoga question? Because it reflects a misunderstanding by many well-meaning people about what it's like to live in chronic pain.

It falls in the same class as other questions: "Have you tried heat and/or cold?" "My sister-in-law swears by massage; want me to ask her about it for you?" and "I hear good things about acupuncture, so have you ever thought about that?"

Duh. Chronic pain sufferers probably have thought about that. A lot. All the time. A long-time chronic pain sufferer has likely tried a dozen treatments. Believe us, no one has thought as much about how we can get relief as we have. No one is more attuned to what might make life less miserable. No one has been more possessed to find promising treatments than we are.

Sometimes able-bodied people who have no experience living with the kind of pain we endure show a bias. For them, chronic pain is a problem to be solved. For them, it's a cipher: Break the code and it's done, over, finito.

But for those of us who have chronic pain, it is not about healing. It is a condition to be lived with, coped with, managed. While there are exceptions, for many serious sufferers a complete cure will not come. It's unlikely that we'll be returned to total health the way someone would be if he or she broke a leg, got a cast, and waited until the bone knitted, soon to be totally fine.

CHRONIC PAIN HARMS LIVES

Chronic pain is different from a condition to be resolved. It's enduring hurt whose intensity tends to take over lives.

For folks like me, chronic pain is, in fact, a separate

disease distinct from whatever injury or illness first caused it. In 2024, it was accepted as such by the International Association for the Study of Pain (IASP) and codified in the International Classification of Diseases.

This means chronic pain can become its own syndrome. The brain gets conditioned to feel pain, even when the injury or illness has healed. The body becomes overly sensitized to pain.

WHAT SUFFERERS REALLY WANT

Even the question "How are you feeling?" is fraught.

No matter how well intended, most often we interpret it to mean "Haven't you solved your problem yet?" "Are you getting better soon?" or even "Are you done whining so we can move on?" That embarrasses us and shuts us down.

Even though it's often difficult, we'd love to talk about our condition with you. We're willing to open up. What we really want is to be listened to and, most of all, to be understood.

So, an inquiry into how we are feeling, as in "What are you going through at this point in your life?" is welcome as long as you want to invest the time in a genuine conversation. The distinction is admittedly subtle, but it's real.

Chronic pain is terribly lonely and isolating; you cannot experience my pain and I cannot experience yours.

It helps if we can share with others and talk about what we are going through, what we feel, and what help we need.

So, instead of asking "Have you tried yoga?" consider engaging in real discussion that gets beyond the idea that we are something to be fixed.

select ... treatment with exercise, multi-disciplinary rehabilitation, acupuncture, or mindfulness-based stress reduction. The guidelines also strongly recommend, based on low-quality evidence, several mind and body approaches including yoga.

Neck Pain
There is some evidence that yoga may provide short-term improvements for neck pain.

Headaches
There is some evidence, based on a few randomized controlled trials, that yoga may improve the intensity of headache pain and may help reduce frequency and duration of headaches.

Arthritis
Results from clinical trials suggest that some mind and body practices, including yoga, may be beneficial additions to conventional treatment plans for patients with arthritis, and some studies indicate that these practices may do even more to improve other aspects of patients' health than to relieve pain.

Listen. Really listen.

Have you tried that yet?

Pain Points

"Strange as it may sound, some people get overwhelmed when they hear about other people's pain. Offering quick-fix solutions seems to be their way of coping."
—Klaus J. Schmitz

Pain Points are comments on this essay as it appeared originally on Medium.com. They are solely the opinions of the commentators and do not necessarily reflect the views of the book author or publisher.

26

Inevitable Pain, Optional Suffering

*A "biopsychosocial" approach to chronic pain
is better than mere medicine*

"I'm leaving," my counselor told me during one of our last Zoom sessions.

Damn! I thought. *What am I going to do now?*

Over the previous year or so my therapist, a licensed clinical social worker (LCSW), had gotten to know me better than anyone ever has. I shared my innermost thoughts, feelings, and secrets in the hope of achieving "peace of mind," the goal I gave him. We had worked hard on cognitive behavioral therapy (CBT), basically talking through feelings so that the insights gained affect how I think and act.

We particularly concentrated on easing my chronic pain. I met that counselor through a medical practice specializing in treating pain (which I refer to in this article as a "pain practice") that prescribes the fentanyl patches I use to keep my hurt at bay (see chapter 7). He was on staff, and, therefore, took my insurance. My co-pay was $35 per session, a bargain price to see a mental health professional.

Each week we would meet in person or via video and delve into the deepest feelings I have about my pain and my experience as a husband, father, and retiree.

> *"We would meet ... and delve into [my] deepest feelings."*

We developed a relationship based on trust. He helped me work through what I've experienced, physical and emotional. He opened my thinking about my chronic pain and my life, but most of all he was someone to talk with to get my feelings off my chest, to complain, to plan, to share, to commiserate, to unload, and to just talk about stuff.

195

Make Biopsychosocial Services a Part of Your Treatment

If you (or loved ones) suffer from chronic pain, here are some tips for building a biopsychosocial approach into successful treatment:

Ask your pain practice if it has a mental health professional on staff or can provide a referral
My sense is that not many pain practices are enlightened enough to offer therapists, but a few do. If that is the case with the one you see, take advantage of the opportunity. Or, as an alternative, ask the doctors you work with for a referral. They may know a mental health provider experienced in treating people with chronic pain.

Search your insurer's database
If you absolutely need to use insurance, turn to your insurer's online database of mental health providers, which can be filtered by specialty. I've found it tough to find someone that way, but it might work for you.

Search for a therapist on *Psychology Today*
The magazine's website offers a database of providers who may be able to help you. You can filter for things such as gender, specialty (including chronic pain), ethnicity, insurance taken, and so on.

Over time, we made progress on my pain. I began to see the roots of my pain running deep into my psyche and experiences as far back as my childhood. We never had a big made-for-TV epiphany, but we made steady progress, and I felt better.

I knew he was paid to talk with me, but our relationship felt closer than just transactional. We'd established a sense of professional intimacy that I had not experienced with a half-dozen or so counselors before.

And then he was gone.

PUZZLED REACTION

I was puzzled. The only explanation I got was that he and the powers that be at the pain practice disagreed on the direction of its psychological services and therefore he was leaving his job. That left me and several other patients out in the cold.

I use this story to introduce the importance of treating the whole person, not just the symptoms, when it comes to chronic pain. Before then, my pain practice had recognized that chronic pain is complex and goes beyond physical injury. It involves many factors, including social and psychological.

Chronic pain, research has shown, is a miswiring of the brain that becomes unrelated to actual physical injury. In other words, chronic pain really is all in your head (see chapter 15). Therefore, how you think, the experiences you've had, and the relationships you've formed all play a role in how you experience enduring hurt.

By having a mental health professional on staff, the pain practice had taken what's called a "biopsychosocial" approach to pain, which has been shown to yield superior relief compared to merely treating physical problems with medicine or procedures.

Research has found that totally focusing on medication and procedures is often inadequate when helping patients cope with chronic pain. Enlightened pain physicians understand that better results can be had by taking a holistic approach to pain.

WHAT IS "BIOPSYCHOSOCIAL"?

A common quote, often misattributed to the Buddha, goes, "Pain is inevitable. Suffering is optional."

(According to One Mind Dharma, "… [T]he earliest known attribution is in 1983 to Karen Casey. Some sources also quote Haruki Murakami … a prominent Japanese author [from his 2007] book *What I Talk About When I Talk About Running*.")

Tracey Chester, founder of and a therapist at the Pain Trauma Institute in San Diego, is writing a book on pain and trauma. (See Pain Profile: Surfing for Relief.) She agrees pain and suffering are two distinct things.

"There is pain and there is suffering," she says. "The 'bio' portion of biopsychosocial is there for the physical pain, the psychosocial part is to ease 'the suffering.'"

The biopsychosocial treatment model integrates biological, psychological, and social factors in understanding and treating illness, Chester explains.

It recognizes that health and disease are influenced not only by physical or biological factors but also by a person's emotions, behaviors, social environment, and cultural context (see chart next page).

Then email a few to see who is taking on new patients. Don't hesitate to get on a waiting list, if that's available. Many providers offer free "get-to-know-you" sessions. I found my current counselor this way.

Consider private pay
Some mental health providers simply don't want the hassle of dealing with insurance companies. They may be more likely to take you on if you are "private pay," that is, you compensate them directly.

This can be expensive but may be worth it in terms of really getting to the roots of your pain. And your bills may be reimbursable if you file claims with your insurance company.

Factors	Focus	Treatment Approach
Biological Factors	Involves physical and physiological aspects affecting health, including genetic predispositions, anatomy, biochemical imbalances, infections, injuries, or physical ailments	Medical Interventions such as medications, surgery, physical therapy, or lifestyle changes (e.g., diet, exercise).
Psychological Factors	Includes emotion, thoughts, behaviors, personality, and mental health conditions that influence the well-being, considering factors like stress, coping mechanisms, and beliefs about illness.	Therapies like cognitive behavioral therapy (CBT), stress management techniques, mindfulness practices, or psychiatric medication when necessary.
Social Factors	Involves interpersonal relationships, cultural background, socioeconomic status, and support systems, with influences from family dynamics, work environment, social support, and cultural beliefs.	Interventions such as family therapy, social skills training, community support programs, or addressing barriers like poverty or discrimination.

Chart courtesy of Tracey Chester

Adds Chester:

Technically, a biopsychosocial approach includes taking medications and having medical procedures. This is the 'bio' part. However, pain does not occur in a vacuum. It happens to a human being and affects all aspects of life, hence 'the psychosocial.'

The Society of Behavioral Medicine offers this example of how the mind and body interact when it comes to chronic pain:

[P]ain catastrophizing, defined as the tendency to magnify, ruminate, or feel more helpless about pain is associated with worse pain outcomes including greater pain intensity and interference. Mental health providers can play a key role in helping individuals cope with chronic pain by reducing pain-related negative thoughts and increasing an individual's overall level of physical exercise and engagement in value-based activities.

PATIENTS ARE BEING SHORTED

If chronic pain sufferers get only medical care for chronic pain, they are being shorted. Pain is less likely to be relieved if treatment ignores the psychological and social. Mental health comorbidities are common for those of us in pain.

A 2025 study published in the JAMA Network Open showed, for example, that around two in five adult chronic pain sufferers also have serious depression and/ or anxiety. The study's authors wrote: "To address this significant public health concern, it is essential to routinely screen for mental health symptoms in clinical settings where people with chronic pain are treated."

Other research has shown that treating the whole biopsychosocial person yields greater results than simply medicine alone. Chester cites an article from a 2007 *Psychology Bulletin* that concluded the following:

Interdisciplinary pain rehabilitation programs (IPRPs) based on the biopsychosocial model lead to:

- *Better pain reduction and increased physical function compared to traditional medical care.*

- *Higher return-to-work rates: Studies show 63% of chronic pain patients in biopsychosocial programs return to work, compared to 24.5% in conventional treatment.*

- *Lower healthcare costs and medication dependence: Functional restoration programs reduce opioid reliance and healthcare utilization.*

Too few pain practices recognize the psychological and social connection to chronic pain. Chester feels they should employ therapists to help patients better cope. Unfortunately, few do. Patients are left on their own to piece together biopsychosocial services elsewhere:

> *"Too few pain practices recognize the psychological and social connection to chronic pain."*

Having psychological services in a pain practice is an enlightened way of treating people in pain. It recognizes the reality that chronic pain is as much mental as physical and that treating it involves treating the whole person.

MY SEARCH FOR A NEW COUNSELOR

The pain practice I attended used to be one of those enlightened providers when it came to taking a biopsychosocial approach to pain treatment, but it is not anymore. It hasn't replaced my counselor, and the physician assistant I deal with to get my medication doesn't know of any plans to do so. The practice has gone through ownership changes, and the mental health aspect apparently isn't a priority.

I think the execs who run the practice chose to concentrate on prescribing drugs and doing procedures, which make the company (and the execs) more cash than does providing psychological services. But clearly patients like me need more holistic help. I'm not sure the decision-makers know all the good that my counselor did for patients like me. Do they care?

> *"The state of mental health access in America is atrocious."*

My counselor's leaving the pain practice kicked off my yearlong search for someone to replace him.

The state of mental health access in America is atrocious. There are just too many people searching for too few therapists, in part because so many people need help coming out of the pandemic. It's doubly difficult to get someone who takes insurance.

I searched my insurer's database for a psychiatrist, psychologist, or LCSW to see, but the information it provided wasn't helpful. I couldn't find any providers close to my home or that were taking on new patients. I also wanted to see a man, which cut down the candidates more. I called my insurance company for help, but all its representative did was refer me back to the online search.

I finally took some advice from Tracey Chester, who recommended the *Psychology Today* website. I clicked on the database links Find a Therapist and Get Help for a provider specializing in chronic pain in my home area.

I emailed five; three got back. One looked like a good match. I started to meet with him in 2025, and our trust grew. Still, it was discouraging to have to redo all the work I'd done with my previous counselor. Also, he doesn't take any insurance. He is expensive (at $180 per hour), but I do get some reimbursement.

I had to search long and hard for someone to take a comprehensive approach to my chronic pain when my counselor left. It was, frankly, harder than it should have been.

My journey to find mental health help is an example of how difficult it is to build an entire biopsychosocial approach to chronic pain, particularly with someone experienced in that model. I'm grateful that I'm getting the help I need to deal with all aspects of my pain.

Don't shortchange yourself when it comes to coping with chronic pain. Seek out the full range of services you need to cure your hurt.

Pain Points

"It is remarkable how the therapist's farewell becomes more [negatively] charged than the pain itself. Perhaps this is an indication that true suffering is not in the pain, but in the stories surrounding it?"—Peerspective

"Saying that pain is all in your head is not a radical statement. A truly radical statement is that everything is in your head. This is, in philosophical terms, called Idealism. It goes something like this: Everything we see, hear, taste, touch, feel, etc., is mediated by our brain/mind. We can literally experience nothing except through our minds."
—Gary Buzzard

Pain Points are comments on this essay as it appeared originally on Medium.com. They are solely the opinions of the commentators and do not necessarily reflect the views of the book author or publisher.

27

Defending Demon Drugs

Don't hate the fentanyl and sister medications that make my life and those of millions of others bearable

I use fentanyl every day.

I am physically dependent on it. I rely on it to live my life. I am not an addict.

> *"Fentanyl is 50 times more powerful than heroin."*

Every 72 or so hours, I remove a patch bearing the opioid from a foil package, peel off the plastic sheets protecting it, and stick it to a shoulder, waiting for the relief it will bring. The opioid is 50 times more powerful than heroin and up to 100 times stronger than morphine, says the Drug Enforcement Administration (DEA).

I suffer from intense chronic pain caused by a genetic disease that deforms my joints. As a result, I deal with chronic pain 24/7.

The fentanyl, a synthetic drug developed and used successfully for surgeries since the '60s, doesn't erase my pain. It makes life bearable.

I don't use it to get high. In fact, the time-delay transdermal patch delivers it in amounts small enough (25 micrograms per hour, the second-lowest dose available) that I don't feel any effect other than pain relief. No euphoria, no giddiness, no buzz. I don't abuse it. I use it completely legally.

(Let me again be clear before I go on: I am not a doctor or other healthcare professional, just a chronic pain sufferer speaking from my personal experience. I am not recommending any treatment for chronic pain or any medical condition. Always consult an experienced, informed, licensed physician before pursuing any treatment. Misusing fentanyl can be fatal.)

The problem is that fentanyl and sister opioids such as hydrocodone, morphine, and oxycodone are heavily stigmatized (see chapter 33), a hangover from the days in the early 2000s when some doctors handed out pain pills as though they were Skittles.

Because of this, legal users like me are sometimes dismissed as addicted drug seekers by policymakers, physicians, pharmacists, family, friends, law enforcement, and the public.

We are collateral damage in the war to end the "opioid epidemic." (See chapter 18.)

AMERICA'S SCOURGE

Fentanyl and related opioids have certainly been a scourge on America, responsible for a rising number of overdose deaths over the past three or so decades. According to the CDC: From 1999–2021, nearly 645,000 people died from an overdose involving any opioid, including prescription and illicit opioids.

Recently the rate of deaths has actually decreased: "Provisional data from the CDC's National Center for Health Statistics indicate there were an estimated 80,391 drug overdose deaths in the United States during 2024 — a decrease of 26.9% from the 110,037 deaths estimated in 2023." Whether this is a trend or a blip is still unknown.

The main culprit in recent overdoses has been fentanyl. Reports *Statista*: In 2021, around 70,600 people in the United States died from a drug overdose that involved fentanyl.

These kinds of scary stats caused alarm among the public, politicians, and policymakers. One of the main ways they responded was to cut the supply of pain prescriptions and pills. It seemed logical: the fewer drugs available, the fewer deaths, right?

Except it has not worked out that way. As supply of prescriptions between 2012 and 2022 was reduced, deaths soared, meaning that the strategy of cutting supply is a failure.

The CDC reports that the opioid epidemic morphed over the years, unfolding in three distinct deadly phases: 1. legal pill prescriptions for OxyContin (falsely marketed as nonaddictive) and other opioids in the early 2000s; 2. illicit heroin in the 2010s; and 3. illegal fentanyl from 2013 through today.

So, there has not been just one overall opioid epidemic, but a series of them, each with its own challenges.

THE OPIOID BATTLE

The battle to limit opioid deaths has been fought over decades.

One response to the first phase — the prescription pill crisis — was 2016 guidelines from the CDC about using drugs to treat pain. Doctors and other professionals interpreted the guidance as setting inflexible limits on prescriptions they could write.

According to NPR, the result was politicians in state legislatures and governors' mansions cutting access to pain medication. Further, it said, "Doctors grew wary of giving opioids at all, which often led to sudden disruptions of treatment, resulting in physical and mental agony, and even a heightened risk of suicide."

Actions like these caused a backlash, however. Pain sufferers complained that they were unintended casualties in the war on opioids.

Responding, the CDC loosened its guidelines for pain care in 2022 (it took six years of people suffering), in part clarifying that each pain patient should be considered individually rather than being viewed in terms of inflexible rules — and that strict limits on pain prescriptions were not a good idea.

Other efforts to curb illegal fentanyl are ongoing. Millions of doses of Narcan (naloxone), which revives people who overdose on opioids, are being made available everywhere, including through vending machines. Narcan nasal spray has been approved by the Food and Drug Administration (FDA) for over-the-counter (OTC) sales.

"I don't want to downplay the danger of opioids."

I keep naloxone beneath the sink in my bathroom. In many years of using opioids, I have never come close to administering it. As I've said, if one could die from slight fentanyl exposure, I'd have passed years ago.

THE PROBLEM FOR PAIN SUFFERERS

I don't want to downplay the danger of opioids. Those hundreds of thousands of overdose deaths over about two decades are tragic. I feel for the families of those who passed. But the focus on cutting the domestic supply of opioids has created artificial shortages of pain meds. In 2024, in *The New York Times*, anesthesiologist and pain medicine physician Shravani Durbhakula wrote about the current struggle to get drugs patients need:

> *[My mother-in-law's] medical condition quickly deteriorated, and her pain rapidly progressed. No one questioned that she needed opioid medications to live with dignity. But hydrocodone and then oxycodone became [in short supply] at her usual pharmacy and then at two other pharmacies. … [Her] care team required in-person visits for new scripts. Despite being riddled with painful tumors, she endured a tortuous cycle of uncertainty and travel, stressing her already immunocompromised body to secure her medications.*

> *"The pendulum has swung too far the other way toward prohibition."*

> *My mother-in-law's anguish before she died [of pancreatic cancer] in July 2022 mirrors the broader struggle of countless individuals grappling with pain. … They do not understand why [my husband and I], doctors whom they trust, send them on wild goose chases. They do not understand how pharmacies fail to provide the medications they need to function. They do not understand why the system makes them feel like drug seekers.*

Back in the early 2000s, prescription abuse clearly drove the opioid epidemic. Now, however, the pendulum has swung too far the other way toward prohibition.

FEAR AMONG SUFFERERS

In my research for this book, I joined Zoom support sessions by the U.S. Pain Foundation and Facebook groups of chronic pain sufferers (see Sources of Solace).

The folks I've encountered are frustrated and scared. The Facebook forums are full of comments — particularly from women (see chapter 19) — about not being taken seriously by doctors, pharmacists, and, often, family. Posters complain about being denied insurance coverage for drugs, about how expensive drugs are without insurance, and about how physicians and pharmacists sometimes refuse to write or fill prescriptions, seemingly arbitrarily.

Why? Doctors, pharmacists, manufacturers, and insurance companies have been burned. Some pill-pushing physicians have been jailed for overprescribing. Big Pharmacy companies like CVS and Walgreens and drugmakers like Johnson

& Johnson and McKesson have agreed to pay a total of $54 billion for damage caused by irresponsible distribution of pills (they admit no wrongdoing). No wonder they are gun shy about opioids.

The government has work to do to crack down on doctors who write unnecessary scripts, but the most urgent problem today (in the third phase) isn't legally prescribed fentanyl and other opioids, it's *illegally* manufactured, trafficked, and distributed drugs leading to hundreds of thousands of overdose deaths. The ingredients for those mainly come from China and the products are made and distributed mostly by Mexican cartels.

Over-restricting legal prescriptions and supply punishes everyone — including physicians who provide opioid medication for legitimate reasons and, by extension, pain patients — for the crimes of a relative few.

Sure, get rid of the bad apples, but don't withhold the whole barrel.

SICK AND TIRED

Pain sufferers are sick and tired of being shamed and stigmatized for their hurt (see chapter 33).

My pain physician assistant tells me that her practice constantly deals with insurance companies trying to cut off payments for pain medicine. This is not because they don't want to shell out the money; she feels the problem is the stigma of opioids built up over the years. Insurers and others in the chain of pain care treat situations such as mine as though I am in acute pain, which eventually goes away with treatment, rather than chronic pain, which, for many sufferers like me, is a never-ending condition.

From the Facebook and Reddit support groups, I get a sense that people are despondent over their chronic pain. Some appear fed up and suicidal. (If you are thinking of doing self-harm, call or text the 988 Suicide and Crisis Hotline at 988.)

There are many tales of lives ruined by pain, of deep grief over the mostly hurt-free lives they've lost.

Others complain that family, friends, healthcare providers, and insurance companies label them as liars about their pain, druggies seeking highs, and people who drone on and on about their conditions.

There is moral condemnation at work. Those who don't have constant pain — like many policymakers, physicians, and members of the public — see pain sufferers as wimps, as not tough, as having failure of character. Some leaders believe people in severe chronic pain should just step up, take individual responsibility, and not complain.

This frustrates pain sufferers. As an example, here is a typical post from one on Facebook:

> ## "Doctors give me this look of disapproval and suspicion."
>
> *How do you deal with being treated like a drug addict? I hate asking for pain medication because of the stigma around it and just about all doctors give me this look of disapproval and suspicion. I end up in the emergency room for debilitating pain fairly often and though I have a diagnosis of a chronic illness that has a key characteristic of excruciating pain, I never feel listened to. Even my primary care doctor has started to want to deny my pain medication. I try to explain that I understand I am young and it is a last resort with risk of addiction, but [I] feel the benefit outweighs the risk because without pain management, I miss out on my education, income, and socializing, and I struggle with everyday tasks such as cooking, cleaning, and showering. I bring pictures and documentation on my flares and still my doctor treats me like I frivolously take pain medication.*

MY PAIN-RACKED BODY

The consensus is that multidisciplinary approaches to chronic pain work best. Treatment might include physical therapy; cognitive behavioral therapy (CBT); interventions such as shots, stimulators, and implants; alternative therapies such as acupuncture; and more.

I've tried most of them with little relief.

These therapies have their place, but so does medication. In this context, think of fentanyl and the like not as illicit drugs but as medicine to treat real people in distress from actual accidents, conditions, and illnesses.

My individual situation, in which my entire body is racked with pain, makes fentanyl the right choice for me. Other pain sufferers have their own personal circumstances to cope with. It should be caring, educated physicians, in the context of ethical practice — not politicians — who decide what best helps us as individuals. Overall, we need a more nuanced discussion about opioids for pain.

DEFENDING THE INDEFENSIBLE

How can I defend the indefensible, the demon drug fentanyl and its sister opioids? Isn't it foolish to think that some of it isn't necessarily the scourge everyone thinks it is?

Yes, there have been hundreds of thousands of tragic deaths from opioid abuse. Yes, even for legal drug takers, there is always a danger of addiction. And yes, getting off these drugs and going through withdrawal is terrible. There's no question that caution about opioids is warranted.

But the operative word is *caution*, not *prohibition*.

I am terrified about what would happen if I couldn't get my fentanyl prescription. Not only would I deal with severe withdrawal but living with the pain that the drug masks would be unbearable. That sounds dramatic, I know. (Pain sufferers are often accused of being overly dramatic.) But it is the truth. People without constant, debilitating pain don't get it.

Like most things in life, fentanyl is not purely good or evil.

In the wrong hands, it kills. In the right ones, it heals.

Pain Points

"After ... trying to help [my] patients with chronic pain for almost 50 years, I've come to several conclusions. Number one: I'm glad I'm now retired! Number two: just like a diabetic who needs insulin or people with heart conditions who need their medication to maintain their heart rate and blood pressure, there are many patients suffering with chronic pain who need their medications to improve their quality of life! There is a vast difference between addiction and dependence. [That] is not understood by the majority of people, including physicians and pharmacists. ... People who are dependent on medications to improve their quality of life should never be judged as addicts or drug seekers, but [they should be] shown respect and compassion for their courage to go on!" —Dennis Hatfield

"I'm not a sufferer of chronic pain, but even in the instances I've had acute pain in recent years (for example, surgery, broken bones, etc.) it was hard to get sufficient pain medication to effectively see out the pain period. I felt that the doctors were more concerned that I'd become addicted to pain medication than they were about my pain and suffering at the time. It does no good to tell them I don't get addicted, because they either don't believe me or don't care. I cannot imagine how difficult it is for someone with chronic pain to deal with the system!" —Fiona Shearer

"The campaign against fentanyl is so absolute. Also, I'm biased because my dad was a painkiller addict. I honestly don't know if his situation was one of real pain or addiction. … No one should suffer permanently when there are solutions available." —David J. Elrod

"Chronic pain patients are victimized by the opioid epidemic. After seven spinal surgeries, I'm getting tired of the battle. Recently, my pharmacist let me know that after five years of my using his pharmacy, he can no longer fill my opioid pain medication because independent pharmacies are facing additional scrutiny. So, now I start over because no big box pharmacy will fill the scripts. … I feel nothing from my medication except less pain. I've done the same research. … Overdoses on the rise while prescribing declines. How long before they realize chronic pain patients with legitimate prescriptions aren't the problem?" —Dena@Write-Solutions

"I don't like the existence of fentanyl because prior to its widespread existence those unfortunate enough to succumb to the lure of street drugs weren't in so much danger as today. Of course, the easy solution would be not to go to the dark side, and everyone knows it. Still, a lot of regular, normal people in our society will try illegal substances at least once in their lifetime. … It's weird how the same thing can be a lifesaver for some who desperately need help, and a death sentence for others who equally desperately fall into the depths of personal hell of substance abuse." —Asper

Pain Points are comments on this essay as it appeared originally on Medium.com. They are solely the opinions of the commentators and do not necessarily reflect the views of the book author or publisher.

PAIN PROFILE

Surfing for Relief

A pain sufferer and therapist harnesses
nature, exercise, and community to ease hurt

Tracey Chester believes that surfing soothes the body and soul.

So much, in fact, that it's integrated into her practice as a therapist and counselor of chronic pain sufferers.

As the founder of the Pain Trauma Institute in San Diego, Chester works with others locally to organize surf therapy sessions aimed at giving participants relief from their grief, trauma, and pain. She harnesses the power of nature, body movement, and sport to shake up the many feelings that come with enduring hurt. Chester tells me:

"Surf therapy has all kinds of benefits."

> Surf therapy has all kinds of benefits. It is a powerful, holistic approach to managing chronic pain and trauma. It offers hope and empowerment to people navigating these challenges. It fosters physical strength, stress relief, and emotional release while building resilience and self-confidence. Participants also gain from a sense of community and peer support, reducing feelings of isolation often associated with chronic illness.

Chester took up surfing when she moved to San Diego in the mid-2000s. "I'm not a great surfer and never was," she admits.

GETTING THE IDEA
One morning in 2019, she saw an interview on *Today* with another local, Natalie Small, who runs a nonprofit called Groundswell Community Project and does ocean therapy around the world. They connected to offer surf therapy outings in their hometown.

Recently, they hooked up with a professor at the University of Southern California who received funding to study whether surf therapy actually works. The test group was small, only nine people, but results of the research showed that getting sufferers out on the water positively affected their pain.

The research measured how participants felt before and after surfing based the McGill Pain Index. It isn't the usual 0 to 10 pain scale (see chapter 21). Instead, it presents assessment takers with words that describe pain. Pre-surf, each participant selected words that described their pain, such as *wrenching, stabbing, cramping, sickening,* and *burning.* The data was collected and presented in a word cloud; the more times a word was selected by a participant, the bigger it appeared. The results for pre-surf showed 270 words, with the most common ones being *exhausting, throbbing, aching, tight, hurting, sore* — all negative terms. Post-surf, participants chose two-thirds fewer words, meaning there was a significant decrease in pain. Chester reports: "The word 'exhausting' turned to 'tiring,' which is a completely different version of the same symptom. Of course, you'd be tired after surfing. The word reflects a more positive meaning of the feeling."

The USC study hypothesized surf therapy works because it is an immersion event, like cold plunging. But it also has a slight threat of danger from being out on the waves, which concentrates the mind and body to work together.

"You have to pay attention," Chester observes. "You are in a dynamic situation with some degree of danger, which could be a wave knocking you down. You need to be aware of sea life in the water."

PLAYING IT SAFE

Chester adds, though, that surf therapy is not paddling patients far out in the water and having them ride big waves. The sessions are 70% on land and mostly about learning about the ocean, finding out about themselves, and creating community. Each person has a surf safety team member who rides on the back of the board, which are for beginners, close to shore. Participants learn gradually over the 4-to-8-week group sessions.

She says: "Thus the 'threat' part of the immersion is there but not overwhelmingly, as safety is crucial. Some days, a patient might choose not to go in the water because her body is not up to it."

The 56-year-old adds that the experience of surfing with others, including many women she calls "surf sisters," creates a state of mindfulness that is hard to duplicate elsewhere. Chester says:

For many participants, surfing therapy became a turning point in rebuilding trust and confidence in their physical abilities. They found themselves gradually pushing past their fears. One person experienced joy for the first time in years. Laughter and play are important; as adults, we don't play enough. When someone stands up on the surfboard for the first time and can't believe she's done it, it's amazing. There's no feeling like it.

MIND/BODY CONNECTION

After working several years as a geologist, Chester changed careers at age 38. She became a certified clinical trauma professional, a licensed marriage and family therapist (LMFT), surf therapist, and a certified grief counselor because of decades of pain.

She's had severe neck pain, thyroid issues, headaches, and problems with her left big toe. Most of these required surgery and medications, including opioids. Further, she had endometriosis that had been undiagnosed for decades and caused extreme pelvic pain. In September 2024, she underwent a hysterectomy, with the hope that it will solve her abdominal problems.

Chester says that her pain was caused by much more than damage to her body. In 2022, she attended a webinar by Gabor Mate, MD, author of books including *When the Body Says No: Exploring the Stress-Disease Connection*. She had a revelation: her pain linked to childhood trauma. Early on her parents told her they had decided to get pregnant again because her older sister, Liza, was dying of brain damage and Chester would be her replacement in the family.

"As I grew up, I was told that the only reason I was born was because of her," says Chester, who adds that Liza is still living. "But my chronic pain and trauma of the family's dysfunction are inexorably linked."

WINDOWS OF TOLERANCE

Chester describes what she does as "trauma-informed therapy." She works with patients on managing their "windows of tolerance."

"Her pain was caused by much more than damage to her body."

Most people in pain have small windows because they hurt so much. At best, the pain is distracting; at worst, it's mind-clouding agony. Get outside those windows of tolerance and people become hyperactive on the one hand or shut down on the other. Chester's patients stretch their tolerance zones to create spaces where they can do a better job of remaining calm, thinking clearly, and managing stress.

Before founding the Pain Trauma Institute, Chester worked as a therapist in a physician's office and saw a difference between how patients spoke to her and what they said to the doctor.

She recalls: "Patients would talk to me, and they could tell me all their feelings. When they got to the doc, they would literally shut down and not be able to say anything."

> *"Most people in pain have small windows because they hurt so much."*

Chester draws a distinction between the physical, which a medical doctor might address, and the mental, which a therapist like her can deal with. Patients should have access to both (see chapter 26).

Chester has more of a mission than just exposing her clients to the healing waters off California. Her goal is nothing less than reforming healthcare to address the whole person — body and mind — when treating chronic pain and other conditions.

She fancies herself as a "medical translator" between how patients talk and how providers communicate. She's writing a book on medical gaslighting and trauma, aimed at women dealing with the healthcare system. (Chester uses the word "gaslighting" in the sense that some providers inadvertently dismiss patients' symptoms as merely psychological, rather than addressing both the physical and the mental.)

> *I am on a crusade to integrate both, to educate physicians about the importance of having therapists in their practices. Medical schools don't teach doctors that having therapists is a great idea. To help chronic pain sufferers and others, we need to address both the body and mind.*

CHESTER'S ADVICE

Based on her personal and professional experience and expertise, Chester advises chronic pain sufferers like her to be proactive in managing their care:

Bring an advocate along to physician appointments

> *Don't ever go in alone. Go with somebody who can communicate well and take notes. You need someone to ask pertinent questions of the doctor.*

Communicate to doctors what you can't do because of your pain

> *Tell them what you do for work and how the pain limits you. Say, 'I'm a lawyer*

(or an accountant) who can't practice because I lose my train of thought from the pain' or 'I'm a teacher (or a salesperson) and just can't stand up for long periods of time,' something like that. They'll take you more seriously.

Create as holistic a treatment plan as possible

Address every possible piece of your pain, body and mind.

See a pain psychologist

Find a therapist who's not judgmental and can work on your nervous system, which you can learn to control through things like heart rate variability, neurofeedback, somatic experiencing, hypnosis. There are a variety of such procedures that can help as well as the medical piece.

Treat yourself as you would treat someone else

Give yourself the compassion you deserve. Too many people say, 'I'm weak,' 'I don't deserve help,' or 'I'm a burden.' These thoughts get in the way. Self-blame really undermines any progress a person can make.

Understand the science of pain

Research the body-mind connection so that you know pain is not all in your head, the way we are sometimes led to believe. Learn about pain science and childhood trauma.

Take care of yourself

Allow your budget to include self-care. I hear a lot, 'I can't afford massages.' I say, 'Can you afford to fix your car?' I want you to think of yourself as a car. I'm not saying to go bankrupt but start looking at your expenses and spend more on yourself. You deserve it.

28

Hurt Feelings

I interviewed dozens of sufferers and experts to learn about the anger, guilt, grief, and other common emotions that come with constant hurt

I feel guilty every time it happens.

I'll be in my La-Z-Boy listening to my wife tell me a story about how her cousin is trying to deal with her husband, who has Lewy body dementia. I'll sit there trying to take in all the information, but my body is searing with head-to-toe hurt.

As my wife and caregiver, MeK, continues to speak, I try to hide how I feel, but my face betrays me. I look grouchy, grumpy, and gruff.

"Are you mad at me?" she'll ask, sensing that something is amiss and wrongly assuming that she did something to piss me off.

> *"I try to hide how I feel, but my face betrays me."*

I am in searing pain as I sit there. As much as I try to focus, the discomfort distracts me from what's going on around me. I just can't concentrate.

As I wrestle with how to react to my wife, inside I am a mess of emotions. I'm worried about how long it will take the pain to pass, if it ever will. I am ashamed at seeming weak, too weak to "man up" and tough it out (see chapter 20). I am guilty for making my wife feel bad, realizing she knows something is going on with me. I am angry and just want to scream. So, I just shut down.

I muster all the energy I can to answer her question. "No. You didn't do anything wrong," I tell her. "I hurt. I just need to sit quietly right now." This kind of interaction embarrasses me. Because of the pain, I am not myself. My negative emotions take over. I experience the maddening swirl of mind-body connections that make up my chronic pain.

This is a vicious feedback loop for chronic pain sufferers: Our pain affects our emotions and our emotions affect our pain.

For this book, I've done extensive research into chronic pain, including interviewing dozens of sufferers and experts. Among the questions I ask: "What are the most common emotions chronic pain sufferers feel?"

Though the answers could have been all over the place, there was remarkable consistency among sufferers and experts as to what feelings chronic pain causes.

Here are the seven most-common emotions of chronic pain (in alphabetical order), with perspective from people I've talked with.

ANGER/RAGE/FRUSTRATION

Anger and frustration are part and parcel of each other. Sufferers often feel trapped by our circumstances and this leads to feelings of rage.

I become angry sometimes when I see others walking across the parking lot or in a store and not experiencing any pain or difficulty. I wonder why I can't be like them. Why do I have to be impaired? I get angry when I am in pain and I become difficult to get along with. My husband frequently shows me compassion and I regret getting short with him. —Terry F., Knoxville, Tennessee (people who prefer not to use their last names are identified by first name and initial.)

"When your body is constantly in pain, the body itself can begin to feel like a source of danger."

Sufferers often look for fault, and sometimes that turns inward toward self-blame or feelings of, "what did I do to deserve this?"

Women, in particular, often get mad because they are gaslit by doctors (see chapter 19).

In the days before I got diagnosed (it took me over 15 years to get a diagnosis and associated treatment), I felt a lot of anger toward the healthcare system as a whole. Gynecologists and general providers dismissed me and told me that my symptoms were nothing out of the ordinary and something I'd just have to live with. —Brittany Ferri, Newark, New York

ANXIETY/FEAR/WORRY

Chronic pain is a beast. It's wild and unpredictable, leaving sufferers in a constant state of alert, hypervigilance, and "dis-ease" (see chapter 6). It causes a fear in the short-term ("Will my next step or standing up hurt like hell?") and long-term ("Will I always feel like this?").

Patients fear that pain will get worse, or that their fears about the future will come true. Patients can be fearful of losing their job, fearful of not being able to take care of themselves, fearful of not being able to take care of loved ones, or fearful of not being able to enjoy activities they love. — Kevin Huffman, DO (doctor of osteopathic medicine) and board certified bariatric physician

Fear makes sufferers feel unsettled and even in danger.

When your body is constantly in pain, the body itself can begin to feel like a source of danger. Life turns into something to be braced for or against, rather than enjoyed and lived. A lack of a sense of safety and connection with your essence (self, mind-body, intuition) is the single greatest determinant of lingering pain. —Justin Krull, registered physiotherapist and co-owner of Myofascial Canada, Mississauga, Ontario

There is always fear that the other shoe is going to drop, the fear that a day will come when there is nothing to be done but be in pain. —Rebelle Summers, chronic pain sufferer, digital nomad, and writer

DEPRESSION/DESPAIR/HOPELESSNESS

Chronic pain and depression are common companions (see chapter 10). After trying all kinds of treatments that don't bring much relief, sufferers can become despondent, leading to despair and hopelessness.

Many of my clients seek therapy when they are at a very low point. They may have struggled to connect with others, may have very few answers for their condition, may have to live with pain flares, and may struggle to keep up with the responsibilities of being a functioning adult. Accompanying this lowness is often a sense of hopelessness, not just about finding symptom relief, but more so about experiencing joy and meaningful relationships. —Cynthia Shaw, PsyD, licensed clinical psychologist

There is also often a keen sense of loss.

I felt intense, physical suffering and agony in my back and my neck. I also had all-over body pain from fibromyalgia. The mental suffering I felt was depression and anxiety over my inability to live the life I had expected or planned. —Stacey P., Bryan, Texas

And, sadly, depression and despair can lead to thoughts of self-harm and suicide.

> *I have suffered from depression for almost all my life. When I have a pain flare-up, I have suicidal thoughts. I wish the pain could end.* —Berenice Frazer-Gale, Ipswich, Suffolk, England

(If you are in the US and feeling suicidal or thinking of self-harm, call or text the 988 Suicide & Crisis Lifeline at 988.)

GRIEF/REGRET

Grief is among the strongest emotions we chronic pain sufferers feel. We mourn our old lives and future ones that are never to come.

> ### *"Grief has been my constant companion."*

> *I still grieve my former life. Back home in Maine with my sister recently, we talked about the changes that life had brought my way, especially leaving my job in a school district. And suddenly it all overcame me and I began to cry. What I experienced was akin to the death of a loved one. I literally went from having a job I loved, a job that made each day fun, to unemployment. I now realize that just like losing a loved one, this grief will weaken over time. But it will never go away.* —Mark Harrington, Dallas

> *Grief has been my constant companion. I don't mourn my old life, only for the one I would never get to live.* —Rebelle Summers

It can be the everyday simple things that sufferers regret.

> *I miss my old life when I'm working in my garden because I can no longer do the things I used to do and brought me joy. I can no longer get on my knees and plant a row of bulbs or flowers because it is too painful. I so miss my old life.* —Terry F.

Some sufferers experience the classic Elisabeth Kübler-Ross stages of grief, but not in any particular order.

> *While the stages of grief (denial, anger, bargaining, depression, and acceptance) are somewhat applicable, the emotional journey in chronic pain can be cyclical and iterative rather than linear.* —Jason Polk, counselor and the owner of Colorado Relationship Recovery, Denver

Some people feel grief is good.

I have gone through a state of mourning about the 'old me,' but I have let that go. I have come to accept where I am at this point in my life. I think we might need to go through a grief period. It's healthy to acknowledge that you aren't the same person you were. —Roz Potenza, Tampa Bay

GUILT/SHAME

Guilt is a heavy burden for pain sufferers. We feel shame at being disabled and for the toll that pain takes on our families.

I do have guilt, for what I have cost my wife. Her life would have been much different if I hadn't had a stroke. I logically know that there is nothing I could have done to prevent it, but I still feel guilty. —Jim Ferrone, Flemington, New Jersey

Sometimes I feel guilty for being a burden. Everybody says to me 'You're not a burden' but when people help you so much, it's hard not to feel a little guilt. And then I always wonder could I have done something that would have prevented this. I know that's insane thinking. But I'm human. And maybe I'm insane. LOL. —Mark Harrington

Feeling too much guilt can sour relationships with family members, friends, and others.

Addressing this guilt that people with chronic pain often feel regarding the perceived burden they place on their loved ones is crucial because it can significantly impact their relationships and overall mental health. —Joni Ogle, licensed clinical social worker (LCSW) and a certified sex addiction therapist (CSAT)

Constant pain is exhausting. I struggle to sleep. I get headaches and I have had to change my plans to fit my pain levels. Every day my pain is different. I want to be a calm, level-headed wife, mother, and friend, but pain makes me cranky. I feel guilty a lot for not doing things with my children or family and friends. —Berenice Frazer-Gale

Guilt comes from different places, including the idea that we shouldn't feel that way.

Because I don't physically look disabled, I sometimes tend to gaslight myself so that maybe it's not as bad as I'm making it out. My guilt is especially prominent when I prioritize rest. That there are so many other things I 'should' be doing even though I know I will trigger a flare or burnout if I entertain those internal demanding voices. —Rebelle Summers

LONELINESS/ISOLATION

Pain is extremely lonely (see chapter 16) because we each have an individual, unique experience of it. As I've said elsewhere, you cannot feel my pain and I cannot feel yours.

> *It can be lonely having loved ones who can't possibly know what this is like.*
> *—Jacob Kendall, Fairhope, Alabama*

> *When my pain is high, I often isolate until I feel better. That's not always a great idea. My doctor has told me that no matter what, I must keep moving even if it hurts. Isolation is depression's cousin, and I will not let either one overcome me.*
> *—Stacey P.*

Many times, pain brings an intense sense of "otherness" (being apart from or unlike other people).

> *It's common for chronic pain to lead to feelings of sadness and isolation. Many patients withdraw from activities and social events because they fear making their pain worse or feeling misunderstood. —Taher Saifullah, MD, founder of Spine & Pain Institute Los Angeles*

It hurts when we have to leave behind our work, social connections, family functions, hobbies, travel, and more.

> *No one can take loneliness away; it's invisible and not well managed. Yes, I think I feel stigmatized because of how unabated and insidious it is. —Susan Hoffman, Frisco, Texas*

Digital nomad Summers remembers that she felt lonely living in pain throughout her entire childhood and early adulthood:

> *I felt broken, but I couldn't let anyone in to see my brokenness for fear that people would leave if I did. That fear was confirmed when I [started] being honest, not because I actually was the burden that I was made to feel I was, but because the version of me that I had to mask ended up attracting many of the wrong people.*

Isolation is a struggle for sufferers of all ages, but particularly the young.

> *This is true especially for those who experience ailments at a younger age and who struggle to keep up when it comes to physical activities. Dating or making friends are challenging enough tasks for anyone; they can be even more*

challenging for those with chronic conditions. There may be anxieties about not being accepted or needing to go through the whole rigmarole of sharing intimate pieces of their lives and enduring possible consequences and unknown reactions. It can become exhausting and lonesome. —Cynthia Shaw

People have said to me that I'm too young [at age 25] to have chronic pain. They compare what they have been through to what I've experienced and then they don't let me talk. I know that I am young, and it doesn't seem that I should be in pain, but I know people who are younger than me who have chronic pain. I try to stay calm but, in my head, I am so mad. —Katie Schweiger, Minneapolis

> *"I try to stay calm, but … I am so mad."*

RESILIENCE/GRIT/OPTIMISM

The emotions associated with chronic pain aren't all bleak. Many of us discover strength we never knew we had. We develop the courage to face up to our conditions and the hope to keep moving forward. Most of all we are resilient and we have grit, the ability to push through problems and remain optimistic.

Those most successful in managing chronic pain tend to exhibit resilience, an openness to … treatments, and a proactive attitude toward managing their condition. —Joni Ogle

Resilience can provide the will to push forward.

Every so often I've been told I'm brave, whether it was moving to New York City at age 19 or writing vulnerably about an experience. But I see those sparks of courage in me as not necessarily about wanting to be brave, but about wanting to be more actively engaged with my life rather than being a passive passenger. I want to know how to make my life more enjoyable and feel worthwhile regardless of what my pain threshold of the day is. —Rebelle Summers

Coping with pain requires plenty of patience. It takes persistence to keep seeking answers despite the challenges chronic pain brings.

I believe resilience and adaptability are two important traits shared by those who manage chronic pain the best. In addition to using meditation or calming methods and being open to experimenting with pain management treatments, those in pain typically have a robust support system. A major contributing factor to their toughness emotionally is their capacity to maintain flexible

minds and concentrate on what they can control rather than what they cannot.
—*Ryan Peterson, MD, NuView Treatment Center, Los Angeles*

Sufferers who are resilient express pride in not letting pain win.

I have demonstrated extreme resilience through these 15 years of disability. I have been a beacon for my friends who are also going through tough times. I believe my disability has made me stronger and wiser. I handle the unexpected with much more grace now than I ever did. —Stacey P.

When my husband talks about my pain, he says I am 'the strongest person he knows.' But I am trying only to get through the day. It feels nice to hear those kinds of phrases. It encourages me to carry on and be strong.
—*Berenice Frazer-Gale*

Pain Points

"People don't understand pain. Not even those [whom] one lives with. I've learned to be happy in my isolation as a reader of books and a listener of music. They keep me sane when the rest of my world and life has collapsed around me." —Rehmat Jamal

"Chronic pain is a shapeshifter. ... Some of the difficulty of invisible illness ... is the expectation that since you look healthy you must be pain- and worry-free. The phrase 'but you don't look sick' is a tremendous trigger for me. It requires a patience I simply don't have most days. I'm busy trying to get done what I can, and to challenge folks' naive ideas of what constitutes a sick body is too exhausting, most of the time. ... That can make me angry. ... Here's to all of us and our losses; here's to all of us and our triumphs." —Jenn Biddle

"[Guilt] is one of the things I know I focus on a lot. I have a lot of 'shoulds' and guilt from how I was brought up. ... I'm learning to release the guilt, but I have to remember it is a process." — Missy O

Pain Points are comments on this essay as it appeared originally on Medium.com. They are solely the opinions of the commentators and do not necessarily reflect the views of the book author or publisher.

29

Mope, Cope, Hope

*I follow a familiar pattern when dealing
with enduring hurt*

I thought I had screwed up my just-replaced knee.

After the operation, I spent nearly three weeks in a rehab facility in Farragut, Tennessee. A couple of days before my release, the pain and noise started. My new left knee felt like it had a "fuzzy" pang (I can't think of a better way to describe it), and it made a grinding sound when I moved it.

I panicked.

Most of my time in rehab I spent alone in my room, with breaks for physical and occupational therapy sessions and meals. I passed most of my time watching TV and fretting. I worried about how the operation went and whether I'd recover well, but mostly about how my life would be as I contended with what could be lifelong chronic pain.

> *"It's hard to explain the depth of despair."*

When the post-op knee pain started, it's hard to explain the depth of despair I felt. Here, I and my insurance company had spent what I estimate to be more than $50,000 on the operation, only to have me mess it up. All the effort to prepare for the procedure, all the doctors' and nurses' time, all the hope I had for relief, might come to naught.

I had the knee replaced just under a decade ago because of the pain from a rare genetic disease that caused my bones and joints to deform as I grew and aged. It was one of a total of eight joint replacement operations I've had plus I had my ankles fused. Nowadays, I suffer from severe osteoarthritis that makes my body ache from top to bottom.

I was convinced I had damaged the left knee during rehab. The head physical therapist pushed me hard. In the last days of my stay, I dutifully did my exercises under his watchful eye. He had a demanding style that reflected his work with mostly able-bodied replacement patients, not people with my genetic condition.

I'd do knee lifts, knee curls, and other exercises designed to strengthen the muscles around my newly installed joint. These hourlong sessions were designed to get me back on my feet and able to care for myself. Being a good patient, I complied with what the physical therapist wanted me to do, no matter how hard it was. I kept telling myself, *I can do anything for five minutes; push through.*

Then, a couple of days before the rehab facility would discharge me, the fuzzy pain started. It persisted as I finally went home and left the physical therapist and his tough-love style behind. I was truly despondent at the thought that wanting to do the right thing by going into rehab might have turned into the exact wrong thing, a major mistake that would leave me in more pain than when I started.

I came to see a pattern with my pain. When faced with a new twist such as that left knee replacement, I go on an emotional journey consisting of three steps — moping, coping, and hoping.

MOPING

There's no way around it: Chronic pain is depressing.

In fact, 40% of chronic pain sufferers have serious depression and/or anxiety, according to research funded by the U.S. Department of Defense.

Chronic pain saps you. It takes tremendous energy. The body is caught in a perpetual fight-flight-freeze mode, always on alert to danger in the form of the next pang or zap.

Chronic pain causes me to mope. I feel hopeless, as though I've been given a life sentence to a prison of pain.

This has happened many times in my pain journey. I've contended with many moments of despair and gotten swallowed in a deep hole of sadness.

The moping stage is necessary. It is when I take an assessment of the situation and see what life will be like as I contend with chronic pain. But it's important that I don't get caught in it, that I find a way out of the sadness. I don't want to get stuck in my pain.

226

Eventually, I dig out of my moping. I cultivate an attitude that says, *I can manage the pain, I can cope.*

COPING

The second step I go through is deciding how to cope with the pain.

Part of this is practical, such as setting up accommodations that help me feel better. It could be as simple as getting a pillow that allows me to sit or lie down with less pain. It can be taking medications, perhaps including opioids, to ease the pain (see chapter 7). Or it can be as complex as having a joint replacement operation — or eight in my case.

> *"I cope chiefly by having a purpose in life."*

I cope chiefly by having a purpose in life. My chronic pain crashed my career (see chapter 4), making me unable to work as a journalist and marketer. I was out of it for more than a decade while I found ways to manage. I did physical therapy in a pool. I had injections. And I have kept myself busy by doing this book.

This is very distracting from my pain — a key form of coping. Getting lost in a profession or hobby helps take a sufferer's mind off the pain. Other forms include everything from mindfulness meditation and online support groups.

Eventually, I find ways to manage my chronic pain and move from merely getting by with my pain to the next phase: hope.

HOPING

Hoping means having a more positive attitude toward my pain. I'm not saying I make my pain a plus; there's no way to do that. It means cultivating optimism that my life can get better with time and effort.

There are amazing things being done to help people in pain. Scientists are working to truly understand the mechanics of how pain works in the body (see chapter 35). New drugs are being developed. Novel technologies and techniques are being deployed. There is ample reason to hope that healthcare providers will soon be able to do more to help those of us in chronic pain.

That's external hope, though. I've worked hard to build internal hope. It's a feeling that my life can improve despite my pain. It's a sunnier outlook that I can live a full life within the limits of my disability.

"It means accepting my life as it is, not how it used to be or how I imagine it could be."

It involves becoming educated about chronic pain and how it works. It means seeing a counselor to focus on the kind of person I really want to be. It means getting out into the world to do as many activities as my body will allow. It means developing a social circle of people to support me.

It means accepting my life as it is, not how it used to be or how I imagine it could be.

I rely on family and friends to help me, but I try to beware of being a complainer. Not every conversation should be about my pain. I choose key moments to share. I let people know whether I want practical help or just want to vent.

WHAT HAPPENED WITH MY KNEE

After leaving the rehab facility, as soon as I could I made an appointment with my orthopedist.

I had to wait a pain-and-anxiety-filled week to see him, but when I did, he assured me that the knee was fine, that it was glued into the bones so tightly that little could happen that would damage it. I was relieved somewhat, but still suspicious and disappointed that going to that rehab facility had hurt me.

By the way, I'm not saying to avoid rehab facilities after joint replacement. They can be crucial parts of recovery and helpful, particularly if you don't have someone to tend to you at home. I just happened to have a stressful experience.

It took several weeks, but in the end the particular pain in my left knee went away as it healed. I felt enormous relief.

Later, I realized that in all of my joint operations there has been a time of panic during recovery when I felt the procedure absolutely didn't work, that I must have done something wrong, that the replacement had disastrously failed. In the moment, it is terrifying.

To get through it, I follow my process: I mope, I cope, I hope.

Pain Points

"Those without chronic pain don't understand the mental load of dealing with it for long stretches, even our whole lives. It really grinds you down. The narrative that those in pain, especially invisible pain, are just grousing and should suck it up is pure ableist BS. My pain started when I was 16 and it took me 34 years to get an accurate and thorough diagnosis (diagnoses, actually). And I'm only now learning how my hypermobility combined with the neurodivergence and being female have created the chronic pain framework I've been building on." —Jenn Biddle

Pain Points are comments on this essay as it appeared originally on Medium.com. They are solely the opinions of the commentators and do not necessarily reflect the views of the book author or publisher.

30

The 5 M's of Relieving Pain

A noted pain doctor's prescription to heal hurt

For many people like me, chronic pain can be a pain in the … uh … everywhere.

We ache. We're stabbed. We burn. We're pricked. We feel pins and needles. We have flares. We hurt. We suffer.

In my case, my chronic pain is due to severe osteoarthritis throughout the body caused by my rare genetic disease. Other sufferers may have pain caused by any number of conditions: musculoskeletal aging, diabetes, fibromyalgia, and more.

For this book, I interviewed noted pain specialist Andrea Furlan, MD, professor of medicine at the University of Toronto, and author of the book *8 Steps to Conquer Chronic Pain: A Doctor's Guide to Lifelong Relief.* (See Foreword.) Based on her experience with thousands of patients, she has some insights into pain and how to deal with it.

> *"Most doctors aren't very good at treating pain."*

Dr. Furlan observes that most doctors aren't very good at treating pain:

> *Because chronic pain [lasting longer than three months] is different from acute pain [resulting from injury or illness, lasting less than three months], many people, including the medical professionals, do not know how to treat chronic pain. They use the same tools for acute pain to treat chronic pain, and, of course, they will not get the same results. Therefore, people with chronic pain spend years and decades of their lives trying interventions that do not work for chronic pain.*

Chronic pain is widespread, Dr. Furlan tells me, particularly among certain populations. She reports:

Coping With Pain Advice

From my research with experts like Dr. Furlan and my personal experience, here are some things to remember if you are a chronic pain sufferer:

You are not alone
Millions of other people have chronic pain. In-person and online support groups offer information and companionship. (See Sources of Solace.)

You can feel better
As Dr. Furlan recommends, become a student of your pain. A good place to start is with her book, *8 Steps to Conquer Chronic Pain: A Doctor's Guide to Lifelong Relief.*

You are not your pain
It's easy to become consumed with your pain. Keep in mind that you are more than your pain; you have a full life to live. Distract yourself by getting out of the house, seeing plays and movies, and pursuing interests and hobbies.

Find a purpose
Pain is eased when you have a purpose in life, whether that's work, helping others through volunteering, or taking part in family life. Consciously ask yourself: To what do I want to devote the rest of my life?

You are loved
Chronic pain can be lonely and discouraging so it helps to seek support from family and friends. Make your partner,

Women have more chronic pain than men. Older people have more chronic pain than younger people. Children also have chronic pain. Black, indigenous, and gender diverse people face discrimination when it comes to the treatments they receive. People of low socioeconomic status have fewer resources to manage chronic pain.

In her book, Dr. Furlan recommends creating a toolbox of therapies to cope with chronic pain. She writes:

I once met a young woman who had chronic pain since she was a teenager. She counted 102 strategies in her toolbox. She said she doesn't have a toolbox, but a full-size garageful of tools. Not everyone needs 100 tools in their toolbox. ... [I]t is useful to have at least one tool from each of the five groups.

Dr. Furlan calls these groups the "5 M's:"

MIND-BODY THERAPIES

When it comes to hurt, the body and mind are linked closely. Research — and my personal experience — shows that pain affects emotions and emotions affect pain. It's a two-way street that requires attention to both, the physical and the psychological. But some people refuse to recognize the need for treatments such as cognitive behavioral therapy (CBT). Dr. Furlan comments:

People who do not see the connection [between mind and body] are constantly looking for a quick fix, the magic pill, the other doctor who will discover what is wrong. ... These patients are the ones who do not get better.

MOVEMENT

Motion is medicine, Dr. Furlan believes. Although chronic pain often makes you want to slow down, movement ultimately keeps it at bay.

*'Movement' is more comprehensive than 'exercise'.
... [I]t includes any physical activity, even [ones] at
work, going to and from work, shopping, playing
with your kids, hanging your laundry on the
clothesline, or doing dishes.*

relations, and close friends
allies in your pain journey.
There are people who love you
and want to help.

MODALITIES

This refers to any number of treatments that relieve
bodily pain. They are as simple as a heating pad for
neck inflammation to small TENS units that gen-
erate an electrical current to interfere with painful
nerve signals.

*When I talk about modalities, I am referring to
physical modalities, that is, therapeutic tools such
as temperature, pressure, light, sound, or
electricity,. Heat and cold are excellent temperature
modalities. (I also include orthotics and ergo-
nomics under modalities, although they are not
really a physical modality.)*

MANUAL THERAPIES

Masseuses, physical therapists, and some specialized
machines use pressure on muscles and joints to
relieve hurt. Dr. Furlan believes that massage and
other types of manual manipulation can cut pain.

*Manual therapies involve some sort of hands-on
therapy, or the application of pressure to the
body using a ... device. The three major types of
manual therapies are massage, mobilization, and
manipulation.*

MEDICATIONS

Dr. Furlan prefers treatments other than drugs
for chronic pain that's created in the brain, after a
bodily injury has healed, called 'nociplastic' pain.
She allows that medicine can be helpful and necessary, but urges caution:

All drugs have side effects and all of them lead to some changes in body functions. It would be much better not to take any medication, but that is unrealistic for some patients.

I don't recommend that patients read the list of all potential side effects that can occur with drugs they are taking. That can trigger anxiety and a psychological reaction that causes your brain to make you think you are having all the side effects that you read about in the drug monograph. This is what we call the 'nocebo' effect. Nevertheless, it is important that you mention your concerns to your pain team.

"Pain patients need multiple providers."

I asked Dr. Furlan who should be part of a such a pain team. She says pain patients need multiple providers, including a physician who understands the difference between acute and chronic pain, a mental health provider (see chapter 26), a rehabilitation provider, a social services provider, and a personal coach, who could be a person with lived experience of chronic pain.

"What's the single most important thing a pain patient should do?" I followed up. She replied, "Learn about chronic pain. Be the expert in pain neuroscience."

Dr. Furlan has made a career out of helping people in pain. She has a personal connection to the hurt her patients feel:

I had debilitating menstrual cramps for many years during my teenage years and as a young adult. When I was in my 40s, I had two episodes of debilitating low back pain. And when I turned 50 I had a terrible experience with shingles. I do have myofascial pain in my upper back. Fortunately, I do not have pain every day.

Dr. Furlan concludes:

What motivates me is that I have helped thousands of people with chronic pain to regain their joy.

Movement Is Medicine

*A physical therapist and pain sufferer offers
insights into curbing chronic pain*

During breaks as a physical therapist assistant, Jen Rosenzweig can be found on the mats doing vinyasa yoga.

It's a type of exercise in which practitioners flow from position to position, controlling their breathing and building strength and stability.

Her routine as she works at a PT clinic in the Philadelphia suburbs isn't simply to keep in shape. It's just part of the self-care she does to curb the mysterious chronic pain that makes her life unpredictable. She never knows what pain the day will bring.

Still, Rosenzweig is determined to deal with her pain. As both a physical therapist and a chronic pain sufferer, she has unique insights about coping with enduring hurt.

"I feel as though my muscles are suffocating."

PAIN ALL OVER HER BODY

The 41-year-old, who lives with her husband in a row house in the city, says she feels pain all over her body.

Daily, it is like an achy stiffness. She has rigid forearms and quads. "I feel as though my muscles are suffocating," she says.

On occasion, Rosenzweig adds she gets a cold burning sensation that feels like wearing an Icy Hot patch. A few times a year she has sharp pains in her hips, back, and sometimes neck and right shoulder. She also has pain from concussions caused by two fainting episodes, and she has occasional tremors. Unfortunately, doctors have yet to find an explanation for why all this is happening. One disappointing appointment caused frustration:

Since then, honestly, I've been a little bit frozen. I'm normally very diligent about trying to figure out what's going on, but it's been about three years of searching and now I'm doing it all myself. I am not functionally impaired. Because I have the background and knowledge as a PT, the doctor said there is nothing she could do for me. She told me, 'Yes, you have something. I see it,' but basically blamed it all on my anxiety.

Rosenzweig self-treats her symptoms with yoga, steady state cardio (a moderate, intentional effort), weight training, heat, and rest. She has coped with her pain, she says, through "consistency with workouts, grace, and flexibility in my routine, open-mindedness, and monthly check-ins with a mental health professional."

Her favorite treatment is using a sauna. "I kind of cook myself. It's my way to raise my circulation without movement and focus on my breath and heal my body."

FROM INTERIOR DESIGN TO HEALTHCARE

Rosenzweig came to physical therapy relatively late. She was an interior designer until age 35, when she pivoted to healthcare because she had wanted to help people her whole life. Before she decided to change careers, she was burnt out and stressed from the work environment she was in.

"Now, I love what I do and I have such a better work/life balance. I can focus on my needs and have the time to listen to the signals my body is giving me."

A turning point for Rosenzweig came when a relative had a massive heart attack.

Sitting in the waiting room waiting to hear if he made it through, I thought about the cardiovascular illness in my family, about how my family member really just did not take care of himself, and how my genetics put me in an uphill battle. I decided to take my own health seriously. I thought, I don't want my family ending up in this waiting room scared out of their minds, so at least let me do what I can to mitigate the damage.

For years, Rosenzweig had watched this family member not take care of himself but blame everyone else for his ailments. She sees what that does to loved ones.

I really do believe that you are responsible for how to handle things. You can be miserable and let this defeat you and blame everyone else, or you can feel crummy yet take control of what you can control.

Listen to your body and give it what it needs, whether that's rest, gentle exercises, calm breathing, and other things that help you relax — as well as strength training or cardio. I do all of these. But sometimes you can't do the hard stuff. There are days when you have to take that L."

The most important element in her routine that she has done is to "down regulate," which means to decompress from all the activity that goes with modern life. "Humans are not meant to have so much flying at us at one time," she says.

> "*Humans are not meant to have so much flying at us all the time.*"

ADVICE FOR OTHER SUFFERERS

Rosenzweig's advice for other sufferers: Check in with yourself and learn how to tune into your body to know what it's telling you. She does this by shutting her eyes and scanning herself mentally.

Movement is medicine. Doing nothing typically doesn't solve anything, so movement can help you feel better. The hard part is figuring out what movements and what level of intensity. Maybe it's a quick stretch or breathing technique. Maybe reduce the intensity of your workout that day or modify to an easier position. Maybe change your plan altogether. Do something to get some blood flowing. I always feel better after I move a bit.

Rosenzweig says the worst part of chronic pain is the chronic mental fatigue, anticipating, and trying to figure out what and how her body will react to activity. "I remember telling my neurologist (who agreed with me), 'It shouldn't take five workouts in three days to feel mildly okay at baseline.' But I do it, because the alternative is much, much worse."

Rosenzweig prides herself that she has the resilience, curiosity, and courage to figure out what's wrong with her.

Some days (few and far between), I feel defeated, angry, and overwhelmed. One of my best friends said, 'I'm angry for you,' knowing that I take care of my health better than anyone she knows and still I struggle. It's daunting knowing that I have to manage my condition for the rest of my life with the possibility of getting worse. It's hard not to think that your body is failing you. Luckily, I'm pretty determined not let this thing win.

She concludes: "It helps to take charge of your condition, instead of feeling that it's taking charge of you."

31
Be a Pain Warrior

Seven ways sufferers fight for relief

Pain is personal.

It is unique to each person. It can be described as aching, stabbing, burning, sharp, dull, and more. There is no way, however, to say that my pain is just like your pain, because you cannot feel what's going on in my body and I cannot feel what's in yours.

For this book, I've spent hundreds of hours researching, including interviewing pain sufferers, attending online support groups, joining online forums, reviewing websites, and reading studies, news stories, and other articles.

I've learned a lot about how to battle pain and be what sufferers often call themselves: *Pain Warriors.*

These are people who confront their pain and fight to find relief. Here are seven ways to be a Pain Warrior:

> *"What sufferers call themselves: Pain Warriors."*

BE EDUCATED

Ignorance is not bliss when it comes to dealing with chronic pain. The first step is to learn, learn, learn. Don't be afraid to ask questions of doctors and other healthcare professionals.

Discover how pain happens in the body and brain. Research the different kinds of pain:

- "Nociceptive" is pain due to body damage that usually heals in three to six months

- "Neuropathic" is pain because of damaged nerves.

- "Nociplastic" or "Neuroplastic" is chronic pain that persists after an original injury or illness has healed.

Become a student of your condition. Beware, though, of quacks and scam cures that are prevalent on the Web.

I recommend starting with these books about chronic pain:

- *The Way Out: A Revolutionary, Scientifically Proven Approach to Healing Chronic Pain* by Alan Gordon with Alon Ziv, which talks about how the author and his team developed a technique for curing pain by focusing on brain retraining

- *8 Steps to Conquer Chronic Pain: A Doctor's Guide to Lifelong Relief* by Andrea Furlan, MD, PhD, who has created a process for coping with pain (see Foreword).

BE PREPARED

Enter doctors' visits with a plan. Write down what you want to communicate about your pain and rehearse before your visit. Be specific and use the language you've learned from becoming educated.

I sometimes get nervous about whether I'll get to say everything I want in the short time the physician is in the exam room. Occasionally, I'll print a note about my symptoms and ask the nurse to add it to my chart.

Be straightforward when you talk with docs. Keep to the facts and avoid getting emotional, even if you are desperate to be seen and understood.

Research what might be wrong with you but avoid suggesting a specific diagnosis — it's the doctor's job to do that, and you likely don't know as much medicine as he or she does.

And always take notes in a phone app or notebook, either during the visit or immediately after, of what the doctor said so you can follow up during the next visit.

Sadly, chronic pain sufferers often have to go to a variety of specialists to get the right diagnosis — keeping well-organized, written records can help clear up confusion later. It helps to becomes friends with the doctors' office portal, where pertinent information will be posted after your appointment.

Also, remember you are legally entitled to copies of your medical records, including doctors' notes, if you request them.

Unfortunately, if you are female, doctors may take your pain less seriously (see chapter 19). Some women recommend bringing a friend or relative along to appointments, which may help you deliver your message fully and clearly or at least give you someone who can take notes.

BE PERSISTENT

It often takes a long time to get a proper pain diagnosis, particularly if there isn't an immediately apparent physical reason. Some diagnoses, such as fibromyalgia, are settled upon after eliminating other possible causes — and that takes time (and money). The pain sufferers I've interviewed, however, consistently encourage their peers to never give up. No matter how frustrating your pain journey, there is hope if you persist. It's easy to get discouraged when things drag out for months or even years. Push forward until you get the answers you need. Some people finally find relief after decades.

> *"Pain sufferers ... consistently encourage their peers to never give up."*

BE ASSERTIVE

Speak up when it comes to your pain. Doctors may dismiss you if you don't advocate for yourself. Avoid becoming too emotional and don't be accusatory, but do not be afraid to assert yourself.

I try to be firm, but not obnoxious. Being seen as "difficult" turns off doctors, nurses, and other caregivers (see chapter 24), but I find they'll respect you when you make clear, consistent, and compelling points about your condition.

This takes hard work and it's especially challenging when you feel like crap from pain. It pays off, though, in more accurate and quicker diagnoses.

BE CURIOUS

New developments in chronic pain care happen all the time, some revolutionary and some not so much. Researchers are hard at work on new interventions, medicines, and techniques for treating enduring hurt (see chapter 35). If one seems to apply to you, don't hesitate to ask your doctors about it, though be aware that it takes years for new treatments to be approved by the FDA or other regulators.

Consider signing up for studies of experimental drugs or other treatments available in your home area. (Disclaimer: I am not a doctor. Always check with qualified physicians before submitting yourself to any medical procedure.)

I've set up Google Alerts for the term "chronic pain" that each day tell me about the latest breakthroughs. I also get moving and inspirational stories from other sufferers.

Some advice: Don't focus just on physical cures; also investigate ones that center on the social and psychological aspects of pain, such as brain retraining (see chapter 26). As I advised when talking about becoming educated, beware of quack theories and experts on the internet.

"Don't just focus on physical cures."

BE A PARTICIPANT

One of the best coping strategies is to share what I feel. Seek out local or online support groups, like those by the U.S. Pain Foundation or Chronic Pain Anonymous (see Sources of Solace). Fellow sufferers on these forums are warm and welcoming to newcomers.

Sign up for Facebook or Reddit pain groups and read about others in similar situations. Share and ask questions if you feel comfortable. Interacting with other people is healing.

Many sufferers get help from counseling by psychologists and social workers. It's difficult to find someone who takes insurance, but a close relationship with a professional can put your pain in perspective.

Find a friend or family member to talk about your feelings with. Sometimes, however, those who are able-bodied can't really understand pain because they haven't lived it. They may also become disenchanted with what they may see as constant complaining. So, pick your person carefully. Choose someone with true empathy and love for you.

BE GRATEFUL

Chronic pain is scary, depressing, and emotional — for everyone. I get solace from remembering all the good things in my life, such as the people who love me: my spouse, my children, my old friends.

Even if things look bleak, seek experiences that make you happy — like hummingbirds outside your window or a hobby or craft that's your passion — and express your thankfulness for them. Be grateful for the good things in your life and distract yourself from the bad.

Wherever you are on your pain path, to be a proper Pain Warrior, don't suffer in silence. There are people out there who want to help you with your chronic pain, including caring doctors and nurses. But you must do the work to find them and communicate about your pain if you wish to find relief.

The advice above has helped me on my personal pain journey. I wish you the best of luck with yours.

Pain Points

"The nerves in my c3 and c4 vertebrae are crushed. My Pain Dr looked at me after my recent MRI, his eyes bulging, and said, 'Nothing we are doing is helping you, is it? Your nerves are crushed.' I agreed. I told him that my neck hurt so much I am not able to sleep anymore. It was the first time he got it. He needed updated MRIs to see the continued degradation to understand. He never took me at my word."
—Tabitha Warren

Pain Points are comments on this essay as it appeared originally on Medium.com. They are solely the opinions of the commentators and do not necessarily reflect the views of the book author or publisher.

32

Prayer and Pain

Does belief bring relief?

I awoke in pain.

After a night of tossing and turning (see chapter 8), the sun came up and I opened my eyes. Immediately, I felt stabs of pain everywhere, but particularly in my chest. It was a sickening ache.

> *"Please God, make the pain stop."*

I knew I wasn't having a heart attack. I'd felt this particular hurt many times before. Still, that made is no less awful.

Lying there, I whispered, "Please God, make the pain stop."

Eventually, I woke up enough to get out of bed. After a long few minutes the ache faded. Whether it was moving or an answer to my prayer, I soon felt better.

"Thank you, God," I said as I started my day.

LOSING MY RELIGION

I am not usually a praying person.

When someone asks if I believe in God, I joke, "I'm a Frisbeeist. (Pause.) We believe that when you die your soul flies up on the roof and you can't get it down."

I mostly reserve prayer for serious occasions, such as wishing safe travels for my family members. But when it comes to my chronic pain throughout my body due to a genetic disease, I admit I've prayed for it to end.

I don't believe that God can hear my thoughts, so I say aloud, "Please, dear God, lord in Heaven, father, mother, friend, hear my prayer. I can't take it anymore."

Then I get through that next day, and the next one, and the next. I don't know whether a higher power is the reason for this resilience, but it's possible.

INCONCLUSIVE RESULTS

Prayer is a universal part of human existence, but can it make a difference when it comes to coping with pain? Research shows an absolute ... sort of.

For centuries, pain was considered God's wrath. According to research summarized on the National Institutes of Health (NIH) website:

> In the Middle Ages, pain was considered a religious matter. Pain was seen as God's punishment for sins, or as evidence that an individual was possessed by demons. This definition of pain is still embraced by some patients who might tell the health professionals that the suffering is their cross to bear. ... Many Hindu believers envision pain as a divinely ordained punishment or resulting from personal actions. In Islam, it can be punitive or Allah's will. A popular Buddhist belief is that suffering is the cost of attachment.

The NIH report continues:

> Spirituality and religion may influence the experience of pain and fatigue. Religious people are less likely to have pain and fatigue according to [researchers]. They obtained data from 37,000 individuals, 15 years of age or older, with fibromyalgia, back pain, migraine headaches, and chronic fatigue syndrome. ... They ... found that those with chronic pain and fatigue were more likely to use prayer and seek spiritual support as a coping method compared to other people. Pain sufferers who were both religious and spiritual were more likely to have better psychological well-being and use positive strategies.

ACTS OF FAITH

In researching this book, I interviewed dozens of chronic pain sufferers.

This includes Maryanne Peluso, who spent eight years as a Franciscan nun in the early 2000s.

She wrote a memoir about that time called *Behind the Tapestry: My Discovery of God's Grace Amidst Chronic Pain and Loss* (available on Amazon). It tells the story of how she had to leave religious life in part because of chronic pain from pudendal neuralgia, which caused burning in her abdomen and lower torso.

Peluso credits her faith for allowing her to live with her hurt:

Pain can be a life lesson in faith and how to live totally dependent on God's grace and mercy. I don't know that I would say that I've actually 'overcome' pain but I manage it now — it no longer 'manages' me. My Catholic faith and my strong, close, personal, and intimate relationship with the Lord have made a huge impact. Without my chronic pain I know for a fact that my relationship with Jesus would not be nearly as strong as it is today; I am more understanding and compassionate towards others regarding their own pain and losses.

"My Catholic faith and my strong, close, personal, and intimate relationship with the Lord have made a huge impact."

Like Peluso, others find solace from pain in prayer. Why does it work? An article on PainScale.com notes:

[P]raying is similar to … meditation and, therefore, provides some of the same benefits. However, the focus of the two practices differs. Meditation shifts focus inward to the breath and the self, whereas prayer shifts focus outward to a god, a higher power, or the universe. However, both practices can lower blood pressure and reduce levels of the stress hormone cortisol. They can also improve mental health and reduce chronic pain levels.

So, the power of prayer may come from a deity, or it may come from shifting focus away from what's happening in the body and more toward the spiritual. The simple act of looking outward rather than inward may distract sufferers from their hurt. Sheer optimism that there is a solution to pain might make one more possible.

Another study reported by the NIH backs this up:

Preliminary findings indicate that people who are more engaged with meaningful spiritual and religious practices — such as spiritual meditation and prayer — can tolerate pain better; that is, those more engaged in these practices evidence a greater willingness to accept pain than those less engaged in these practices.

NO COMMON DEFINITION

According to the same NIH article, research into the effect of prayer on pain is weakened by not having a common definition of "prayer" to study. Despite that, it reports:

One study with Muslim women who underwent a caesarean section showed that, compared with a no treatment control [group], women randomized to an Islamic prayer condition reported significantly lower pain intensity scores (i.e., the magnitude of the experienced pain) at three hours and six hours after the intervention.

Other research has shown mixed results regarding the relationship of pain and prayer. In an article for Pain News Network, Lynn Webster, MD, vice president of scientific affairs for PRA Health Sciences, and author of the book *The Painful Truth*, observes:

Medical researchers have looked into the effects of religion and spirituality on chronic health conditions, including chronic pain, for many years. The research has produced vastly different results. According to a review of studies in the Indian Journal of Psychiatry, *prayer may contribute to healing, may worsen health, or may make no difference at all.*

> "*More times than I can remember, I've known people in pain to cry out to God for mercy.*"

Webster continues:

More times than I can remember, I've known people in pain to cry out to God for mercy, kneel in silent prayer, cross themselves or finger their rosary, practice yoga or meditation, wear crosses or angel pins or crystals, express a longing for heaven, mention attending religious services, or tell me about their belief in God.

Even religious skeptics who are in pain sometimes pray for themselves or ask others to pray for them.

The simple fact is that most people have a tendency to turn to God and faith when they are in need, including when they are in pain. Along with most other pain specialists, I have come to see this as generally a good thing, because relating to a God or a perceived spiritual reality beyond oneself can affect one's pain experience positively.

[I]f we're interested in what promotes healing for those enduring long-term pain, we can't ignore the interaction between belief and pain.

Webster's point about even skeptics praying when in pain reminds me of the old saying, "There are no atheists in foxholes."

THE IMPACT OF PRAYER

Some sufferers find solace in methods like the Chronic Pain Anonymous (CPA) 12-step program, which includes belief in a higher power (see Sources of Solace). A 2023 online survey of its members assessed CPA's impact. Among the results, respondents experienced:

- an improved sense of belonging (83%)

- improved group support (78%)

- improved mental well-being (77%)

- improved spiritual well-being (73%)

- improved social connections (72%)

- improved physical health (32%).

While these stats don't show causation between spirituality and pain relief, they hint that spiritually based practices may boost psychological and physical well-being.

What about praying for others? Does it help those being prayed for?

Back in 2006, *The New York Times* reported on a study of whether such "intercessory" prayer helped patients undergoing coronary bypass surgery. The research found:

> *Prayers offered by strangers had no effect on the recovery of people who were undergoing heart surgery, a large and long-awaited study has found.*
>
> *And patients who knew they were being prayed for had a higher rate of post-operative complications like abnormal heart rhythms, perhaps because of the expectations the prayers created, the researchers suggested.*

So, the evidence shows personal belief and prayer may help problems like chronic pain, but praying for others may not.

PRAY IT AWAY

Those who believe in the power of prayer argue that it can't hurt, why not try it? But there are times when it goes too far.

One of the attitudes about pain that most offends me is when people who aren't in pain say to sufferers, "Pray it away," as though that is some magical cure for our conditions. In high school, my eldest daughter, who inherited my rare genetic disease, was told that by her classmates.

Such advice is harmful because it puts blame for having a health problem on the individual, rather than recognizing that chronic conditions are nobody's fault.

"Pray it away" implies the problem is personal weakness, and suffering shows a lack of spiritual strength, a deficit of moral resolve, and being on the outs with God.

Believe me: If prayer alone could cure sufferers like me, we'd spend our days prayerfully begging for relief.

> *"Such advice is harmful because it puts blame ... on the individual."*

HIGHER POWERS

I agree that faith in higher powers can help. I understand that those who ardently practice it believe it can result in miracles. It mustn't, however, be the sole thing we sufferers are told to do.

While spirituality may influence pain, I don't think prayer by itself will wipe it away.

Seeking relief also takes action to treat the pain, whether that be traditional medicine, alternative methods such as acupuncture, or newer ones that retrain the brain (see Pain Profile: Cured by Brain Retraining).

Devout Catholic Peluso concurs and advises her fellow pain sufferers:

> *Turn to your faith, whatever faith tradition that may be. Immerse yourself in your relationship with God or whatever 'higher power' you believe in. But also fight for yourself and for your health. Be your own advocate. Educate yourself. Read articles online. Find books about your condition by others who are going through the same things. Seek and keep a good support system. You have a life to live; get on with living it. There is 'good life' with chronic pain. It may take some work to get there but it is possible. Just don't ever give up!*

Bottom line: There's plenty of evidence to suggest that prayer and spirituality can have a positive impact on chronic pain.

For many, belief is relief.

I'll add this, though: Go ahead. Pray away. But don't neglect additional, more worldly solutions. Follow the old adage: "Pray but move your feet."

Prayer and persistence can work together to overcome hurt.

Amen.

Pain Points

"I like to see prayer as multifaceted and wide open. To me, if I have intention and am doing something for someone, it is prayer (cooking, painting, writing). If I am aware of something and see God a bit more clearly, to me that is God (holding a baby, sharing a warm embrace). Interestingly, these are the things that are most hard for me to do when my pain level is high."—Michele Cambardella

Pain Points are comments on this essay as it appeared originally on Medium.com. They are solely the opinions of the commentators and do not necessarily reflect the views of the book author or publisher.

33

Stop the Shame

Too many people look down on those of us suffering from enduring hurt

I felt intimidated.

In 2025, I visited my pain doctor and asked him about upping the dose of the opioid I use for my chronic pain because my chronic pain had gotten worse.

To ease it, I'd used fentanyl for decades (see chapter 7). It's a powerful opioid up to 100 times more potent than morphine, in addition to my other medications. I use a patch that slowly releases a small amount of the drug into my system over three days. It's never gotten me high, but it takes the edge off my pain and makes me functional. I've never abused it.

I wanted to increase my opioid prescription because my current dose didn't work as well as it has before. This is common as opioid resistance builds up in the body.

But I was nervous about what the doctor would think of me because there is a strong societal stigma and shame around chronic pain and opioid use, including among some doctors.

> *"I was nervous about what the doctor would think of me."*

Boosting the prescription was not a demand, just an idea. But I was terrified of the doctor judging me as a drug seeker and, more frighteningly, punishing me for it.

I felt a pang in my chest just thinking about it.

MAKING THE ASK
I understand my physician has all kinds of pressures and restrictions on what

Pain Stigma Cures

The stigma around chronic pain is hard to shake. But it is just a mindset, so it's possible to have it change. Here's some advice for altering attitudes about pain:

Treat each sufferer as an individual
You likely know someone in chronic pain because at least one in four American adults is in that group. Rather than view each as a stereotype, say as a drug seeker, get to know him or her individually. See each as a whole person who happens to be going through a difficult experience and needs care and attention.

See chronic pain as a medical condition, not a failing
Don't confuse pain with personal weakness. Pain is not a measure of character. It is not divine punishment for personal sins. It is a medical condition, not a moral failing.

Don't conflate chronic pain with opioid abuse
One of the most effective ways to treat pain is with medicine, including, when appropriate, opioids. Yet, too many physicians, policymakers, and members of the public confuse the issue of what to do about overdose deaths with what to do about so many people in pain (see chapter 18). Disentangle the two and see them as separate health crises, each deserving of attention and funding.

he can do. Doctors have gone to jail for overprescribing. I was afraid of hitting a nerve with him. Frankly, I was scared by the whole process. I also feared my pharmacy might be reluctant to fill a prescription for more fentanyl.

When I finally got the gumption up to raise increasing my dose with the doctor, he seemed stern and skeptical, but he didn't shut me down completely.

He said he wanted to start by boosting how much ibuprofen I take. Then, depending on whether that helped, we could talk increasing the opioid at a future appointment. He added his practice places restrictions on what its physicians can prescribe.

I walked out dissatisfied. The doctor didn't do anything wrong, but I felt put off. Still, I didn't want him to see me as overly emotional and difficult (see chapter 22).

As a result, I haven't revisited the idea of more medication with my prescriber in the past few months, sticking to the dose of fentanyl I've been on forever.

Since my appointment, I've wrestled with whether to go to all the trouble of following through. Doubt crept in. I started to question my own pain — and my own judgment.

I asked myself, *Does my suffering really merit more medicine? Or should I just shut up?*

I'm on the fence about fighting the stigma and pushing for what I need.

PAIN STIGMA IS WIDESPREAD

Such is the force of the stigma around chronic pain.

The situation with opioids is just one of the ways sufferers are looked down upon. Too many people with chronic pain are suffering because they worry about what family, friends, physicians, and others will think, not just about drugs they might take but about a more general stigma of illness and disability.

It's time to dismantle the stigmas surrounding pain and its treatment.

Stigma (defined as "a set of negative and unfair beliefs that a society or group of people have about something") can come from anywhere — family, friends, coworkers, healthcare providers, pharmacists.

It is so widespread that 61% of sufferers have experienced stigmatization from providers or pharmacies related to opioid prescriptions, according to a 2025 survey by the U.S. Pain Foundation (see Sources of Solace).

Further, a 2022 research study included in the National Library of Medicine reports:

Stigma experienced by individuals with chronic pain affects their entire life. Literature identifies multiple dimensions ... including public stigma, structural stigma, and internalized stigma.

Complaints from chronic pain sufferers about being stigmatized are all over the Reddit r/ChronicPain forum. Here's a sampling:

- *People ... want a story. 'What happened to you?' ... [They] seem to be looking to ... put some sort of stamp of approval on your tale of woe. Make a determination of whether or not your 'story' warrants using a cane, getting disability, having a parking pass, or whatever else you use or do to live your life. 'Oh, my great aunt Sheila has ... way worse! She still works every day, you know.'*

Teach others about pain
Most people don't really understand pain beyond their own experience with it, which shapes their attitudes toward others. There is, though, plenty of pain science research that shows acute pain and chronic pain have different biological causes and that the latter is a disease unto itself. It's not a problem to be looked down upon; it's a natural part of being human. The better chronic pain is understood, the lesser the stigma.

Practice compassion
Sufferers don't want to be in pain. They didn't choose it. They'd give most anything to feel better. Listen to what they have to say without labeling them complainers, whiners, or difficult. Give them some grace. Like most all of us, they have problems in life that deserve understanding and compassion.

- *I have to slooooowly and carefully explain this to doctors, if I need to see a new one outside my amazing primary care docs. [I say] 'My usual daily pain is about a 6; so, after 10 years, yes — I look very calm, at a 6. I... am not actually calm.' [It is] even harder to explain to everyday people. Also, 'looking fine' set back my treatment and mental health detrimentally. It took 3–4 years, maybe 5, to get my complex regional pain syndrome (CRPS) diagnosis; after like 15 doctors over the years told me I'm just female; too young; just insane; a drug-seeking criminal; or just dunno... byeee. 'Oh! That'll be $483.'*

- *When you tell someone you have debilitating spinal/nerve pain, and they launch into a lecture about how you 'just need to stretch.' That one irritates the hell out of me!! Anyone with severe spinal pain knows we literally spend half our day all day every day doing stretches, physical therapy exercise, etc. Sorry, but stretching doesn't magically cure your spine.*

PAIN STIGMA TAKES DIFFERENT FORMS

There is an array of kinds of stigma against pain sufferers. Among the most common attitudes they face:

You're a drug seeker. This is the most widespread stigma. It's wrapped up in the maddeningly confusing conflation of the opioid crisis, which has taken more than a million lives via overdoses, and the chronic pain epidemic, which affects tens of millions more (see chapter 18). The demonization of drugs like fentanyl, which has legitimate medical uses, has created a public perception that all drugs are bad and using them for pain is weak.

This stigma also causes pain sufferers who need the most help, such as those with substance use disorder (SUD), to avoid doctors. Reports a Department of Health and Human Services (HHS) Pain Management Best Practices Inter-Agency Task Force Fact Sheet:

> *Only 12.2% of people who require treatment for SUD actually seek treatment. Stigma is found to be a significant barrier, with 20.5% not seeking treatment because of negative consequences associated with their work and around 17% being concerned about negative judgments by friends or community.*

You're weak, a loser. Beyond the stigma of drug seeking, there's a more general attitude that if you can't deal with pain, you are of weak character, even a loser. The American tradition of rugged individualism and toughing out difficult problems creates the myth that asking for help, particularly for conditions that can be as amorphous as chronic pain, shows a lack of grit. Sufferers hear from family, friends, physicians, and others, "You just have to live with your pain," "Boost your pain threshold," "Tough it out," or "Man up." Pain seems to bring out moral judgment about your character as a person.

You're depressed, a worrier, a whiner. All kinds of negative attitudes can accompany people in chronic pain. Rather than being seen as those who have a medical condition and deserve help, sufferers, particularly women, can be dismissed as having psychological problems like depression and anxiety (see chapter 10). Minority groups, including Black people, also tend to be taken less seriously. Because pain can be overwhelming, sufferers talk about it a lot, but after a while others may come to see that as endlessly whining rather than healthy sharing.

> *"Often, chronic pain cannot be cured, only coped with."*

Often, chronic pain cannot be cured, only coped with, but others don't understand why sufferers aren't getting better. They become frustrated and pressure us to "fix" our problems with activities such as yoga (see chapter 25) rather than providing the solace we need. Healthcare workers can become impatient with patients they see as complainers and difficult, but that's just the deep frustration sufferers feel coming through. These attitudes have consequences.

Summarizes the HHS fact sheet:

> *Stigma has far-reaching effects on patients and all those involved in their care. Feelings of guilt, shame, judgment, and embarrassment resulting from stigma can increase the risk for behavioral health issues, such as anxiety and depression, which can also contribute to chronic pain.*

WHY IS THERE SUCH STIGMA AROUND PAIN?

Stigma grows because everyone is an expert in pain — we all experience it — and our personal experience shapes our attitudes.

We may look down on pain and disability because we feel vulnerable — that it may happen to ourselves. Or it may be part of the core human need to see ourselves as special, and to judge others.

Pain is essentially invisible. It takes place in our brains (see chapter 15), and because others can't see or experience it, particularly the able-bodied, they may judge us as lying, faking, or seeking attention.

And public attitudes toward pain have been warped by the media, which features those in pain as drug seekers and villains.

Whatever the reason for stigma, pain sufferers don't deserve scorn. Chronic pain is a burden in and of itself. It makes sufferers feel alone and desperate. It gets exhausting when you ladle shame on top of it.

Give sufferers a break. Don't judge them for their pain. Show grace, patience, and compassion. Save your scorn for real villains.

In short, stop the stigma.

Pain Points

"I think healthcare professionals forget the power of just bearing witness to someone's pain — physical and emotional — and simply believing that it is what the patient says it is." — Elspeth Raisbeck

"My friend is a cancer nurse. She has said, many times, how frustrating it is when people are [treated] for cancer and can't get proper pain meds. Real diagnosis. Real pain. Should equal real pain management."—Roz Potenza

"My favorite anti-response is the challenge that you're doing this whole pain dance for attention — my own mother suggested I could have Munchausen Syndrome ('just a little'). And the complete illogic of that always strikes me: Doing this for attention? From whom, the doctors? Because most of the time we get 10 minutes. From our families? Often, they end up resenting your illness (my ex told me a number of times that he couldn't separate my illness from my personhood, and therefore I must accept his blame). From society? Please. The world wants those with chronic pain to just do the thing — the supplement, the exercise, the therapy — so we can get over it, already. The thought that we'd be asking for care because we just want attention is ridiculous. ... I usually answer this by saying 'if I just wanted attention, I would participate in everything I can't now. I'd not burden my loved ones. I'd have more ease in my relationships. I'd see a movie. So my pain gets me less attention. I hope that helps.' I try to say this in as [gently as possible]. It's worked a few times, but the struggle continues."
—Jenn Biddle

Pain Points are comments on this essay as it appeared originally on Medium.com. They are solely the opinions of the commentators and do not necessarily reflect the views of the book author or publisher.

Cured By Brain Retraining

After being in pain for a quarter century,
this sufferer finally found relief

The first time Fiona Symington rode a bike after working so hard to cure her chronic pain, she felt hesitant.

The 43-year-old resident of Oxford, England, was afraid that after a quarter-century coping with enduring hurt, she wasn't physically fit enough to ride and that her "proper pain," as she puts it, might come back. She'd been well for weeks and was still testing her body in various ways to see whether she was truly free from her symptoms and to find out what her new body was capable of.

She started the ride tentatively. Her muscles already burned a bit as she followed the path from her childhood home to the road. Her knees hurt because she was riding the too-small bike she'd had since age 11, but there was no trace of

> *"This is my second chance at life."*

the debilitating pain she'd felt for so many years. Excitement took over and she silently repeated to herself that she had a healthy body and could push on, a message she'd learned during the brain retraining that cured her.

After about 10 minutes, she stopped in a panic. *What if my pain kicks in?* she thought. *What if I'm not fit enough to get back home?*

"Then I looked into the field next to the road and a whole herd of cows stood staring at me," she tells me. "There was no one else around. Wanting someone to appreciate the moment, I shouted, 'Hello, look at me! I'm on my bike! I am riding my own bike!'"

The cows just kept staring at her. She surveyed the hilly road ahead, lost her nerve, and headed home. Still, this 2019 outing was a significant milestone in Symington's pain journey. Finally free to go outside again and ride, she mulled the many things she'd missed out on during those decades in pain. Now, she's flown in a hot-air balloon and tried snowshoeing, hiking, rock climbing, and ice-skating.

"This is my second chance at life, and because no one knows the future, I try to make the most of every moment," she says.

WHEN THE PAIN STARTED

Symington's pain began when she took a riding lesson at age 10. The pony spooked and took off, and she didn't know how to stop it. Eventually, she fell off and was knocked unconscious. She appeared to have no damage but began in the following weeks to feel pain in her back and legs. About six months after the accident, she awoke in severe pain — and it stuck around from there.

"I remember thinking I would go to the general practitioner and he would tell me there was a strain of some sort and I would recover, but the pain never went away," Symington says.

Gradually, Symington experienced pain in her hips, ankles, elbows, back, shoulders, and sternum. It changed over the years depending on how active she was or how stressed, but she always felt "dreadful" pain. One year it was so intense it felt as though she were on fire. Sometimes it felt like something was gnawing deep in her hip. From childhood through adulthood, she was in and out of hospitals, looking for a diagnosis and help.

"I found it hard to describe my pain to others because it could be so bad," she says. "It altered my personality. I was tired from managing it and often grumpy. I had to work everything around my pain and many times standing or sitting for long was too hard. I spent a lot of time lying in bed trying not to move to get it to calm down. My pain ruled my life."

LITANY OF TREATMENTS

Symington tried dozens of doctors and treatments, with no long-term positive results. In response to severe exhaustion when she was in her 20s (following several viruses), doctors also told her she had myalgic encephalomyelitis/chronic fatigue syndrome (ME/CFS) unrelated to her pain. At various other times, she's been diagnosed with a litany of painful conditions: fibromyalgia, Ehlers-Danlos syndrome (EDS), complex regional pain syndrome (CRPS), chronic pain syndrome, and postural orthostatic tachycardia syndrome (POTS). She's tried a slew of different medications ("which never really worked much") and invasive treatments such as two-facet joint denervations, epidurals, nerve blocks, and something called prolotherapy, which involved injecting dextrose into ligaments to strengthen them, reducing pain.

I also used a TENS unit and a doctor once suggested 'cutting my nerves' although he didn't go into detail as to what that would involve. I did physical therapy, hydrotherapy, and occupational therapy. My mum was desperate for answers so she took me to every alternative practitioner she could think of. I tried osteopathy, acupuncture, faith healing, and reflexology but still nothing worked. No one seemed to know what to do. I worried I would never be well enough to work or have a 'normal' life as an adult because of my pain.

One of the most demoralizing effects of Symington's hurt was that she struggled with relationships. She felt isolated from her friends, who couldn't understand what it was like to live in pain.

> *"I worried that I talked about my pain too much."*

I often didn't have the patience to interact with others. I worried that I talked about my pain too much and, indeed, at times I lost friends because they felt I did. Pain was profoundly isolating for me [see chapter 16]. At worst, I was envious that they weren't suffering in the way I was. My life improved when I met other people living with pain and I could be open with them. We found ways to laugh together and build strong relationships. That helped me keep going.

Symington eventually gave up on trying treatments. Then, about six years ago, she saw an ad for a "brain retraining" program on Instagram. She was extremely skeptical but there were so many glowing testimonials that she felt she had to try it. She decided she was going to give it her all and spend time each day doing the required exercises — and got results within weeks. Others take longer to benefit from brain retraining.

"For a very long time, chronic pain ruined my life," Symington says. "It took away so much joy and opportunity, relationships, and career choices. It stole my hope."

WHAT IS BRAIN RETRAINING?
Symington is exceptional in that she ended up pain-free, and as a member of the brain retraining community, she sees more and more people finding such relief. Most chronic pain sufferers can feel at least a little better by focusing on the messages their brain sends their bodies and vice versa.

261

The basis for brain retraining lies in humans' particular ability to adapt to novel situations. In fact, the brain creates fresh neural pathways when faced with new circumstances all the time, a phenomenon called neuroplasticity. The concept is simple: Like plastic, neural pathways are malleable. The problem: The brain can get stuck in habits and patterns.

> *"Chronic pain itself becomes the disease rather than any underlying condition."*

This is a problem for people in chronic pain, which is pain that lasts longer than three months. After the usual healing time for an injury or illness, the brain can get its signals crossed.

Neural pathways can actually create the perception of pain, absent of any physical problem. Pain can become a conditioned response (see Pavlov's dog, who was trained to salivate at the sound of a dinner bell whether there was food or not) as the body and brain are overly sensitized to it.

Then, chronic pain itself becomes the disease rather than any underlying condition. Some researchers describe this sort of pain as a memory, encoded into the neurological system despite the absence of a real source.

But if the brain can create pain, it can also take it away. That's the idea of brain retraining. The technique concentrates on rewiring neural pathways to recognize that pain is a false alarm, that rather than alerting an individual to damage and danger, it helps the person feel safe.

Obviously, this does not help if there is an ongoing injury to the body, like a cancer, but for conditions that are more amorphous, widespread, or can't be traced to a physical problem, brain retraining can bring relief and even a cure, as it did for Symington.

> *The program I did taught me that once you understand that pain doesn't always mean physical damage, then pain signals can actually be calmed down. Such exercises as meditation, journaling, and 'somatic tracking' — with which you get more mindful about your body — are all fantastic in helping with this. But simply learning about pain science and how pain gets generated is enormously helpful. The way the program explained everything to me got through to me in a way nothing else had before. I was being told my pain was absolutely real but that my brain didn't need to create it anymore. I repeated the brain retraining exercises over and over to create new neural pathways in my brain.*

Symington did a type of brain retraining called Pain Reprocessing Therapy (PRT), pioneered by the Pain Psychology Center in Southern California. Learn more by checking out its website at painpsychologycenter.com, a book called *The Way Out: A Revolutionary, Scientifically Proven Approach to Healing Chronic Pain* by one of the center's leaders, and the Curable app.

Brain retraining showed Symington that the answers to pain often lie within.

> *For plenty of people, pain comes when there isn't really anything wrong with their bodies and it's their nervous system that is trying to express fear or another emotion. I am grateful that if I get symptoms now, I can look inside myself and gauge how safe I feel or what emotions I need to connect with to get my nervous system to calm down.*

LESSONS LEARNED

Symington's been pain-free, except for usual daily exertion, for more than six years. She describes her new life in one word: "Wonderful!"

She lives in a house built in 1891. "I have a small garden that I've transformed into a wildlife-friendly place. It is my sanctuary. I have a small pond and grow dahlias and sweet peas. I also have an elderflower tree and a black currant bush."

When she was in chronic pain, Symington was unable to work, but she is now pursuing a clinical psychology doctorate at Oxford. Long term, she hopes to work with children.

"I feel passionate about making sure that other children have a better experience of being in pain than I did," she says.

She also spreads the word about brain retraining and what it did for her on social media and hopes to start a YouTube series. Her message is that not everyone is going to be able to get out of pain, but everyone can do something that helps them feel a little better.

> *That might be changing their diet or exercise regime. It might mean working on their sleep or their stress levels. Social connection is also crucial. Feeling joy and being with others helps calm our nervous system. Making friends can be hard when you live with pain and particularly if you have lost confidence, but it's always worth trying because there are good people out there who care and will benefit from having you in their life.*

For Symington, the worst part of living with pain was fear about the future.

Her pain was so intense that she constantly worried about how long she could survive. She needed just one person who could say to her, "I believe you are in pain, and I can help you." That would have made all the difference in her life, she says.

"Now I can look back on my pain and see it gave me extraordinary compassion and resilience. I survived 25 years of awful pain, so I now feel I can survive anything."

Symington wants to tell fellow sufferers that they are only human, that worry can show up as anger, so they should keep that in mind if they are struggling with relationships. Reaching out and getting outside support, whether that is from a professional or through a support group, is vital to finding relief.

"Pain is too hard to bear alone," she says. "If you are having a bad time with pain, please don't lose hope. Don't give up. Things can change more than you can possibly believe."

34

The Write Stuff

*Physical and psychological burdens ease
when you express yourself*

There are many ways to cope with chronic pain, from salves to surgery.

Most don't help much, research has found.

The most effective one for me is distraction, getting my mind off the pain by doing something absorbing. For a time, the pain fades into the background.

And the most effective distraction for me has been writing about my chronic pain. It could work for you too.

REWRITING MY PAIN

Chronic pain dominates my life because of my genetic condition that caused my bones and joints to deform starting in childhood and continuing throughout my lifetime.

> *"The most effective distraction for me has been writing about my chronic pain."*

Chronic pain is there in the morning when I wake up. It's there at night when I try — often unsuccessfully — to get to sleep (see chapter 8). It's maddening in its relentlessness. It's vicious. I hate it.

At first, I denied my pain. It's a natural strategy among sufferers. Faced with a problem, we try to shunt it away, to bury it within our consciousness. Our instinct is to resist. That never works. The pain always wins.

But since 2024, rather than suppress my pain, I decided to lean into it. I faced it head-on with the idea that the better I can understand it, the better I can cope with it.

Pennebaker's Prescription

In his book, James W. Pennebaker gives a prescription for effective expressive writing. Here are the steps he advises, with my commentary:

Write about what keeps you up at night
Expressive writing works by allowing you to focus on trauma that is most present in your life.

Write at least 20 minutes a day for at least four consecutive days
This is a proven standard for expressive writing, but it's actually arbitrary. It was chosen because of scheduling for a room for students to work in during Pennebaker's original study. The point, though, is to write for a set block of time for a few days in a row.

Construct a story
Tell a tale about your trauma, with a beginning, middle, and end. It needn't be perfect; everyone's story is messy.

Don't sweat spelling, grammar, and sentence structure
Don't let thoughts like *I can't write well* or *I'm terrible at spelling* get in your way. Most everyone can write something. There is not a right or wrong way to write expressively.

This took the form of writing about my pain and that of others. It's apt because I'm a longtime journalist, retired because of my disability, and writing is my main hobby.

In 2024 and since, I wrote dozens of essays and articles about pain, which form the bulk of this book. I've spent countless hours researching chronic pain, amassing a research file of clips of scientific studies, news articles, and profiles of pain sufferers.

I know pain.

WRITING AS THERAPY

I've written about chronic pain to help other sufferers to feel less alone in their hurt, to help them feel seen, to offer information they can use. I did it because I planned this book about what it's like to live in chronic pain. But mostly I've done it for my own mental health.

For me, writing is therapy.

Writing gets the crud out of my feelings about chronic pain. It allows me to work through different aspects of my awful hurt and put them in perspective. It's a chance to examine the trauma my pain has caused, and to let my emotions out.

I've chosen to do this in public by publishing my writing. That's what a retired journalist would do, to share what he or she learned with others.

But I've also done journaling I showed only to my therapist at the time, thoughts that were personal and revealing, even embarrassing. (The derivation of embarrassment is different, but I've always thought of it as the shame of revealing your naked rear end, or "bare-assing.") This, too, has allowed me to get my feelings off my chest.

It can for you too.

EXPRESSIVE WRITING HEALS

Those who study the impact of writing on physical and psychological pain call getting one's thoughts and feeling off his or her chest "expressive writing."

The textbook definition of that is different from what I do by writing in public. Expressive writing was developed by a scholar named James W. Pennebaker, PhD, a social psychologist who did a landmark experiment back in the mid-'80s. He assigned college students to write about either their intense trauma or trivial experiences for at least 15 minutes a few days in a row.

To his surprise, those folks who wrote about trauma went on to visit the campus health center fewer times than those who wrote about nontraumatic events. He took this to mean that writing healed the group who unburdened themselves, and, he says in his book *Expressive Writing: Words that Heal* (with James F. Evans, EdD), "many [subjects] said their writing changed their lives."

Pennebaker adds:

> *[Expressive writing] can positively affect people's sleeping habits, work efficiency, and ... connections ... Indeed, when we put traumatic experiences into words, we tend to be less concerned with the emotional events ... weighing us down.*

On the other hand, he says, "Not talking about important issues poses a health risk."

In about 300 other studies, the effectiveness of writing about emotions has been proven again and again, Pennebaker reports. It leads to improvements in both physical and psychological well-being. For example, one experiment showed that writing actually increases white blood cells and strengthens the immune system.

Use whatever medium is most comfortable
Write on paper or on a device, whatever works best for you. If your wobbly hands or trembly or stiff fingers give you fits when typing, speaking into a recorder might work. The iPhone Notes app can transcribe your thoughts.

Don't just repeat the same approach each day
The point of writing on consecutive days is to give you a chance to re-examine your story from different perspectives.

Keep your writing private
No one need know what you wrote and, in fact, it's better if you don't share. Destroy your writing if it will upset someone to see it.

Revisit and rewrite several days or weeks later
Expressive writing works best when you go back and think about what you said. This gives you a chance to edit and rewrite with perspective.

Follow a "flip-out rule"
Don't expect to feel better immediately after you write. It's common to feel sad or distressed for a couple of hours. And if the subject sparks a severe emotional reaction, prevent a flip-out by stopping and walking away. Don't damage yourself.

Give yourself time to reflect
After you've written for at least 20 minutes, set aside time to

react to what you wrote. Don't try to fit expressive writing between tightly scheduled activities. It works by evoking emotions and it takes time for you to settle.

For more detailed advice on expressive writing, turn to Pennebaker's book *Expressive Writing: Words that Heal*. Also, consider another work he wrote: *Opening Up by Writing It Down: How Expressive Writing Improves Health and Eases Emotional Pain* (with Joshua M. Smyth, PhD).

Writing can be unburdening. He says:

> *As people write about it time after time, their reactions to the experience become smaller and smaller. Other researchers explain that the benefits of expressive writing come from identifying, labeling, and integrating negative emotions into the broader context of one's life.*

Pennebaker notes that men benefit more from expressing themselves because of their tendency to keep feelings in. In a study he co-authored, one group of angry laid-off male high-tech workers was asked to write about losing their jobs, while others in the same situation wrote about the benign subject of time management. He reveals: "Eight months after writing, 52% of the emotional writing group had new jobs compared with only 20% of the time management participants."

The U.S. Pain Foundation (see Sources of Solace) uses Pennebaker's techniques in its online support group, the Writing Room. The group meets most Monday afternoons to do short writing exercises and share. I've found them welcoming of new members.

THE WRITE WAY

As I said, I'm not exactly doing textbook expressive writing with my chronic pain essays. But unburdening myself in this book has had a positive impact on my pain.

It's the write stuff.

By studying and writing about it, I've faced up to the boogeyman of my pain and found him not as scary as I had before.

My wife says, and I agree, that I am more relaxed about my pain, not exactly at peace, but more accepting of my situation. I continue to work on it, with a counselor, and, as Pennebaker observed, the problem has gotten "smaller and smaller."

It's impossible to ignore or suppress my pain, but the distraction of writing, at the very least, has taken some of the weight off my shoulders.

I am a work in progress. Now, start writing.

Pain Points

"Writing can be such a powerful outlet—like giving your pain a place to rest for a while." — Gazala nabi

"Writing is a distraction — more like steering the neck or your brain to something else." —Diamond Writes

"Writing sets us free. For people like me, who can't yell or shout at others, [I can] give it up through words and that is really satisfying." — Vijaykumar Bhoyar

"I've been writing since I was 13 years old, and it's been my only therapy. I imagine and write and express my emotions and feelings and my principles and opinions through my stories and articles, then I'm way better. Writing can cure you because you put everything inside on paper or on device, so nothing is left inside. It's all out, so this is a way of healing to your soul." —Luna A.

"Indeed, a successful writer can be likened to a healthy man! Writing gives joy, strength, and eases stress in one's life!" — Anya, P.C.

"I've known about daily writing for inner release and getting rid of psychological pain but never thought about it as a tool for other pain." —Ann Buss

Pain Points are comments on this essay as it appeared originally on Medium.com. They are solely the opinions of the commentators and do not necessarily reflect the views of the book author or publisher.

35

New Hope for Sufferers

Fresh research into the causes of and treatments for enduring hurt make me optimistic that the future will bring relief

Chronic pain is a bitch.

It takes over lives and leaves sufferers desperate for relief.

In cases like fibromyalgia, chronic fatigue syndrome (CFS), and complex regional pain syndrome (CRPS), pain may be invisible and apparently without cause, leaving some to question whether it is real. It can cause relationship problems, family tension, and career disruption. It whipsaws sufferers through an array of emotions, including grief, loneliness, and depression.

> *"I'm taking stock of where sufferers like me stand."*

Most of all, chronic pain leaves sufferers feeling hopeless.

As a chronic pain sufferer myself, I am no stranger to these complex feelings.

Over the past couple of years, I've written hundreds of thousands of words about chronic pain, ranging from telling personal stories about my own experience, like accepting my pain (see chapter 36), to talking about big subjects, like the opioid crisis (see chapter 18).

Now, as I write this in 2025, I'm taking stock of where sufferers like me stand. Though our situations feel dire, I actually have hope that new trends and technology mean we will find future relief. I see progress in how chronic pain is diagnosed, treated, and thought about. As I look at the latest pain news, I found some hopeful developments:

RESEARCHERS ARE FINDING THE ROOT CAUSE OF CHRONIC PAIN

Chronic pain is wily.

In some cases, there is a direct cause, something to be treated like a bum knee. In many, though, there are questions as to what prompts it. It may move throughout the body, camping in different places on any given day, at any given moment. It may be a frustrating mystery, a what-done-it?

The exact mechanism of chronic pain is still unknown, but researchers are homing in on the possible roots of how it works. Acute pain is tied to damage to the body; the chronic variety is more puzzling.

Recent research conducted by the University of Aberdeen, Scotland, Academia Sinica in Taiwan, and other international experts showed chronic and acute pain are physiologically distinct — that is, two different conditions in the body. This realization clears up confusion about whether chronic pain is just an extension of acute pain or, as researchers discovered, a disease with its own mechanism.

Scientists are identifying the root causes of chronic pain. A breakthrough study, for example, reported that neuron overactivity in the brain stem could be the source. In ordinary circumstances, these neurons put the brakes on acute pain, sparing a person from the worst hurt. With chronic pain, though, the brakes don't work, prompting an ongoing, out-of-control pain response. This discovery might lead to treatments that restore the body's natural defense system.

Other researchers are working on the theory that some kind of chronic pain could be an autoimmune condition in which the immune system attacks the body. And scientists from Stanford University identified "zombie" cells (old dormant cells that build up with age) as a possible source of pain. Targeting the *Walking Dead* cells with drugs may relieve, or at least help manage, age-related diseases like arthritis, Alzheimer's, and Parkinson's.

The more we know about the true source of pain, the better it can be treated.

SCIENTISTS ARE UNCOVERING PAIN BIOMARKERS

One of the most vexing problems with treating chronic pain is that it is often invisible, biologically speaking. Right now, physicians can only quiz patients about their pain and ask them to assign a number from 0 (for no pain) to 10 (for the worst pain imaginable). This is inherently subjective (see chapter 21). It makes providers nervous because they cannot see the problem under a microscope, in a blood test, or with imaging.

Progress is also being made, however, on the Holy Grail of chronic pain: a biomarker that objectively shows whether a person has pain and how bad it is.

In one study, computer learning (read AI) was used to try to use health data to tell the difference between people with pain and those without. It was able to identify pain patients with about an 80% accuracy rate, which is a step toward more objectively diagnosing chronic pain.

"Progress is being made ... on the Holy Grail of chronic pain."

Other researchers have reported that alterations in muscle tissue may signal back pain. One study reinforced the idea that there are microbiome "signatures" for such conditions as postoperative pain, arthritis, neuropathy, migraine, fibromyalgia, and CRPS.

Yet another study compared patients with myalgic encephalomyelitis/chronic fatigue syndrome (ME/CFS) to those without symptoms. As reported in *Harvard Health*, it found "abnormalities involving the brain, immune system, energy metabolism, blood vessels, and bacteria in the gut."

So overall, I'm encouraged that science is making progress in identifying pain via biomarkers. Thus, chronic pain is becoming more "real" and less likely to be dismissed as a phantom disease.

THE OPIOID CRISIS IS EASING

The opioid crisis is a scourge that has caused many societal problems, including 645,000 overdose deaths from 1999 to 2021.

A less noticed issue is that the opioid crisis has been conflated with the chronic pain epidemic in the public mind (see chapter 18). Legitimate chronic pain sufferers endure a severe stigma (see chapter 33) against those who need such medicines for pain relief. Deaths from opioids have been used as an excuse to set severe restrictions on opioid supply from pharmaceutical companies, artificially limiting what and how much medicine chronic pain patients can get.

Recently, though, there is some encouraging news. Overdose deaths attributed to opioids have plunged. In 2024, an estimated 80,391 people passed away, an approximately 27% drop from the year before and much less than a previous peak of 115,000 annually.

No one is sure exactly why this happened or whether it will last. Some speculate that increased intervention — particularly the widespread availability of over-dose-curing naloxone (brand name Narcan) — and law enforcement efforts are working. Cynics say that those who are most vulnerable have already died and there are fewer at risk.

"The hysteria around ... opioids may wane."

Still, while 80,000 is a huge human toll, particularly for their families, the stats are trending in a positive direction, and not just because fewer people are dying. Another positive step is that the hysteria around fentanyl and other opioids may wane. This could help sufferers who need these medications, but who are afraid to ask for them because they fear being labeled addicts.

I'm hopeful that policymakers will finally recognize that the tens of millions of us in chronic pain can benefit from legally prescribed drugs (see chapter 7). And I hope that physicians will be mostly left alone to do their jobs in the best interests of patients, without fear they will be arrested or sued for providing appropriate care for people in chronic pain. I hope that artificial restrictions on the supply of legal medications become eased, particularly since restricting supply has likely done little to solve the problem. I do not advocate decriminalizing illicit opioids, but I do believe we as a society should take a more mature approach to providing legal medicine to the millions of people like me who need it. I'd like some grace to let us get the medicine we need to feel better.

CHRONIC PAIN TREATMENTS ARE BECOMING MORE INDIVIDUALIZED

Someone told me: "There's not going to be a penicillin for pain."

Some researchers (particularly those working for pharmaceutical companies) are seeking a silver bullet for chronic pain, but because pain is so diverse, they are unlikely to find one. Instead, doctors and other providers should focus on individualized care, on treating each pain patient as unique and tailoring treatment to each.

This includes keeping up with the latest research about how different people feel pain.

For example, a study reported the journal *PNAS Nexus* in 2024 found that men and women experience pain differently, opening the door for gender-specific treatments. A greater percentage of females report chronic pain than males, yet they are more likely to be dissed, dismissed, and gaslit (see chapter 19) by the healthcare system.

Other research has found disparities in how pain is treated based on race and ethnicity. It concluded that non-Hispanic Black and Hispanic patients got fewer referrals to specialist care and lesser opioid prescription rates as compared to non-Hispanic white people. And a study found that though Asian people in the US generally report less chronic pain, that pain gets worse when the person is a victim of discrimination and prejudice.

Increasingly, those who treat pain are asked to take a varied, multifaceted approach to care. Some have called this "deconstructing the cupcake," a clumsy attempt to say that one-size-fits-all solutions usually don't work and care should be broken down into more manageable pieces like physical therapy, medication, psychological therapy, and lifestyle changes (like not gobbling cupcakes).

Penicillin for pain is not coming, but I'm optimistic that customized care can make a difference.

BRAIN PLASTICITY IS BEING RECOGNIZED

Chronic pain is a tango between how one thinks and the pain he or she feels.

The physical influences the mental and the mental influences the physical, in a constant feedback loop.

In keeping with individual medicine, this means that chronic pain should be addressed in a "biopsychosocial" way (see chapter 26). The "bio" refers to the physical. The "psycho" (which sparks memories of a Hitchcock movie) refers to the mental. The "social" refers to the relationships and environment a patient lives within.

Yes, treating the physical is important, but pills, injections, or operations alone won't completely relieve the problem of chronic pain. The other factors that go into it must be considered.

Traditional medicine's "this-hurts-so-fix-it" quest is too simplified for chronic pain. Most doctors want a clear problem to solve; they become flummoxed when it appears there is nothing to be done with a drug or surgery.

And no wonder: Most mainstream docs get little education about pain. Plus, addressing all the facets of pain is involved and expensive, as opposed to embracing quick fixes like prescribing antibiotics.

It turns out that the ways one thinks about his or her pain can increase or decrease its severity. For example, catastrophizing pain makes it worse, and using

"Most main-stream docs get little education about pain."

interventions like pain education make it better. Chronic pain is partly a conditioned response, like Palov's salivating dog, that can be modified.

The brain is where pain is processed and perceived. It can determine if pain is terrible or tame. Because of the brain's "plasticity," it can create pain or take it away (see chapter 15). Altering both conscious thinking and conditioned responses is a promising new avenue for relieving chronic pain.

NEW PAIN TREATMENTS ARE ON THE HORIZON

Physicians are fairly limited in terms of what they can do to address chronic pain. They can send patients to physical therapy. They can prescribe medications; acetaminophen (Tylenol) and ibuprofen (Motrin, Advil) are the first line of defense, although taking them long term can sometimes damage the kidneys or liver. On the other end of the spectrum are opioids such as fentanyl and morphine, which carry a well-publicized risk of addiction and overdose. They may also use drugs targeted to nerve pain like gabapentin (though recent research associates it with a greater chance of developing dementia). Physicians can also recommend invasive interventions such as injections, implants, or operations. These can lead to a lot of pain in and of themselves.

Fortunately, doctors' toolboxes are about to expand.

In early 2025, the Food and Drug Administration (FDA) approved suzetrigine (brand name Journavx) as a new way to treat pain. This is important because it comes from the first new class of nonopioid medications in decades. It targets pain pathways involved with sodium channels in the peripheral nervous system, before pain gets to the brain. Right now, suzetrigine is approved only for acute pain, but similar drugs may be developed for chronic pain.

Elsewhere, a number of new approaches to treat chronic pain are coming.

Duke University, for example, is working on using adenosine, a natural compound in humans, to help manage pain, inflammation, and seizure activity. The University of Buffalo created a new molecule that acts like a targeted anesthetic for up to three weeks without the numbing effects of traditional painkillers. Dalian University of Technology announced that it invented a wearable film that automatically regulates the delivery of heat to painful areas, like a smart Salonpas pad. In other materials news, the folks at Texas A&M have invented a malleable material that can be used for implants that relieve pain versus the rigid ones used now.

THE BOTTOM LINE

Innovation is happening in plenty of areas involving chronic pain, for individual pain conditions and for it as a distinct disease.

It may take years for some of these discoveries and inventions to be commonly used, but they are on the horizon.

My bottom-line message: Don't give up. There are good reasons to hope for relief.

Pain Points

"Unfortunately, I am on many pain groups where even the mere suggestion of [brain retraining] gets people downright indignant. [They think] that doctors are saying it's 'all in their head' and won't even try [it], when it's just another tool for our toolbox. … The brain is such a powerful thing. What we focus on truly makes a difference." — Some days, My mind spills words…I'm Cindy

"When I started my pain journey it was due to an extremely needed hysterectomy. No one wants to believe a 20- to 27-year-old (yes it took 7 years) to have this organ removed. My doctor said the day after surgery 'not to be a hero; ask for pain meds when I needed them.' … I told him this was the best I had felt in years. His response was, 'Wow you were in pain.' And life was great for four years until lupus crept in. It does really suck that you aren't believed. [People say] 'You just want drugs.' No, I would give anything not to need them and I certainly don't 'want' them. I truly am of the belief that chronic pain and autoimmune conditions are caused by trauma. I look forward to the day medicine finds a genetic marker or mutation that can be manipulated."
— Bailys Human

"[Healthcare providers are] not asking the right question. Ask, 'Why is the pain there in the first place?' This gets to the root of the problem. Repressed emotions [manifest] as physical pain until they're addressed. The pain will keep presenting and moving throughout the body to keep us distracted from doing the emotional work. Simple knowledge of this syndrome usually heals or brings immediate relief."—Brian M

Pain Points are comments on this essay as it appeared originally on Medium.com. They are solely the opinions of the commentators and do not necessarily reflect the views of the book author or publisher.

36

Radical Acceptance

I'm learning a superpower to
cope with physical and mental pain

I feel humiliated to be seen in my wheelchair.

On occasion, my wife, MeK, will push me through a noisy crowd exiting a Philadelphia Phillies game in a rush. We'll weave through the crush of people, then come upon someone stopped in our way.

"Excuse us," I'll practically yell, bringing unwanted attention to myself. The folks around us step aside, but seem to stare and, to me, think, "Look at that. He's *weird*."

When something like that happens, I feel the "otherness" that I've experienced most of my life. I try to sink into my wheelchair seat as we make our

> *"I used to walk on my own, albeit with a distinct limp."*

way to the lot where we parked our SUV. Embarrassed, I jump into the passenger seat, while my wife hefts the 25-pound chair into the back.

I used to walk on my own, albeit with a distinct limp. I was able to climb steps, with difficulty. I used to cross rushing streams by stepping on slippery rocks, hike trails in national parks, or stroll cities like Paris.

But beginning more than a decade ago, I couldn't do so anymore because of the complex genetic disease that causes my bones and joints to deform and degenerate with age. I lost the ability to walk more than 100 feet at a time. I use a cane for shorter distances and around the house. It is disheartening. When I'm out in public in my wheelchair, I imagine myself judged by others. Feelings of being defective fill my mind. My stomach churns with shame. I am dis-eased (see chapter 6).

My pain isn't just physical; it's also psychological. My feelings about being seen in a wheelchair is an example of the harshness with which I judge my condition, something common among people who are different from the supposed "societal norm."

I may be projecting, though. Perhaps people around me don't give me a second thought. It may be that they aren't as judgmental as I perceive them to be. It could be that they are more accepting of disability differences than I imagine.

Maybe I'm just judging myself.

For me and others with disabilities or barriers, negative attitudes about ourselves are poisonous. They reinforce the idea that we are rejects, broken, and strange because we have something "wrong" with us.

I'm working to reject this type of thinking in favor of another: radical acceptance.

LOSING THE GENETIC LOTTERY

I've written before: "I lost the genetic lottery" as compared to winners like Tom Brady, Paul Rudd, and Rob Lowe.

I now regret that sentiment. It reinforces a mistaken notion that I've carried since childhood: to be born with a particular piece of DNA is to be a loser. It ignores that all humans are on a genetic spectrum; one variation is not better or worse than another. We can sympathize with (not pity) those in more unfortunate circumstances than ours.

"Acceptance is a gift to yourself." People in chronic pain — whether from genetics, car accidents, or other causes — suffer more than most, but less than many. Others face their own challenges. Life is not a contest to decide who has the heaviest or lightest cross to bear. The point is to accept everybody where they are in life, including yourself, and to provide help for those who need it. This is not so radical an idea (see also: Jesus).

Acceptance is a gift to yourself. It means achieving a truce in the battle between your mind and body. It means shedding the *shoulds* in favor of the *is*. It means recognizing reality without apology.

My toddler granddaughter's favorite movie is Disney's *Frozen*. Any parent of young kids is probably sick to death of "Let It Go," the biggest hit to come out of it. The song has a specific message in the movie, but I see a greater lesson in it. It's an idea that applies to what people with any sort of difference must do. We must let go of our old lives and accept the new as they really are.

ACCEPTING THE RADICAL

Some call this "radical acceptance."

Writes Jennifer Caspari, PhD, a licensed clinical psychologist in Denver, on the *Psychology Today* website:

> *[It] is defined as being willing to fully accept the present moment as it is. Radically accepting chronic pain does not mean you like it or are resigned to it. You can practice tools to improve your quality of life even with pain. Radically accepting chronic pain simply means you completely acknowledge what is happening in the moment without struggling against it.*

As a pain sufferer for more than four decades, Caspari feels as though she is in a battle with her condition.

"[B]y fighting my pain, I am ultimately fighting myself and increasing my distress. Deep down, I know spending my mental and physical energy in a tug-of-war with my pain is futile. It does not make the pain better," she says.

Explains a blog on the website of the therapy and recovery provider HopeWay in North Carolina:

> *Radical acceptance is a distress tolerance skill that is designed to keep pain from turning into suffering. While pain is part of life, radical acceptance allows us to keep that pain from becoming suffering. By accepting the facts of reality without responding by throwing a tantrum or with willful negligence. In other words, it is what it is.*

Radical acceptance can be applied more broadly than just to pain sufferers, of course. It can help anyone who faces life challenges.

Observes clinical psychologist and mindfulness meditation teacher Tara Brach, PhD, in her book *Radical Acceptance*, "The way out of our cage begins with accepting absolutely everything about ourselves and our lives, by embracing with wakefulness and care our moment-to-moment experience."

To accept the radical, sufferers of any kind of pain, physical, or psychological, must drop much of what they assume, that they are broken or damaged people.

They must entertain their own version of the adage, "Pain is inevitable. Suffering is optional." (See chapter 26.)

ACT UP

Acceptance is a superpower. It can be as simple as a personal choice to be at peace with a condition, but it can also be pursued formally through acceptance and commitment therapy (ACT).

Explains an article on HealthCentral: "[With ACT] you practice accepting your distressing symptoms or situation rather than trying to suppress them. You then resolve to make proactive changes in your life based on your values and goals."

Adds ACT patient Kelly Teuscher of Davenport, Iowa, in another entry on HealthCentral:

Every day, situations arrive that are challenging. But I've learned how to deal with various situations and take them for what they are, and this has made my anxiety go down. For the first time, I'm using my mind to deal with my emotions and feelings.

In the same article (by writer Rosemary Black), Beth Dinoff, PhD, a clinical psychologist at the University of Iowa Hospitals and Clinics, compares ignoring pain and its consequences to trying to hold a beach ball under the ocean. It takes tremendous energy and effort. The alternative: Relax and allow the ball to rise to the surface and float. Dinoff says:

Often, people tell me that they just want their pain to go away completely, so they try to push it away as hard as they can. They begin to see how much effort it takes to suppress the negative sensation of pain. Once they have these images of the metaphor, they can apply this to their own lives.

I see a counselor who's using ACT to help me align my thoughts and behaviors with the kind of person I want to be. It's tough sledding. I'm working through decades of conditioning about my pain, my life, myself. It's all part of a "biopsychosocial" approach (see chapter 26) to treating chronic pain that goes beyond just medicine.

PEACE WITH MY PAIN

I've now achieved, however, a kind of peaceful standoff with my physical and mental pain: It tries to ruin my life, and I won't let it.

My days range from bad to less bad; I never know what pain I'm going to get when I wake up. Agonizing sensations to almost acceptable ones come from moment to moment. How I feel depends on the meds I'm on as well as my mindset. I've come to realize that my pain will always be there, for the rest of my time on earth, regardless of what I or my doctors do. It's a fundamental part of my life's story.

By the way, by "acceptance" I don't mean giving up hope of feeling better. Hope is healthy. To visualize a better life and make a plan to get there is also a fundamental part of being human.

But hope and acceptance can coexist, I'm learning.

I maintain hope in part by trying all kinds of treatments, from epidurals to acupuncture to medication and more, seeking relief. Some helped; most failed.

As my body deteriorated and my hurt grew worse, my pain tolerance also improved. Now my chronic pain is a constant buzz in my consciousness, like ringing of the ears. I haven't given up on science or the possibility that something might come along to revolutionize pain care. You never know.

The lesson: Letting go is not giving up.

JETTISONING JUDGMENT

Meanwhile, I'm trying to accept my pain without judgment. It doesn't mean I am broken or bad. I am not being punished. I need to live in the moment and shut out the static that distracts me.

> *"Letting go is not giving up."*

I see acceptance as the path to my ultimate goal: peace of mind. With a therapist's guidance, I'm imagining what that might look like. I'd like to be more at ease with my life, as difficult as that is with my disability. I'm working to escape my conditioning about what is and isn't normal. I'm moving forward toward acceptance in all its forms — acceptance of myself, acceptance of others, true acceptance of what it is to be human.

In the 1960s, Elisabeth Kübler-Ross identified five stages of grief, which others eventually extended to seven. Acceptance and hope make up the final phases. For me, there has been a lot of heartache getting there, but I'm making progress. Hell, I'm practicing acceptance by thinking through this essay. I'm slowly learning to be more comfortable with who I am.

I still get embarrassed by being in a wheelchair, but I accept that it's what allows me to get out into the world. It lets me live my life and "walk" with my wife, MeK.

A woman in an online chronic pain support group I attended put it best: "Acceptance is freedom."

Pain Points

"Since you sound very courageous to me, I'm going to ask you to do something that takes some courage. Are you willing to talk to others, including strangers, and tell them what you want and need at any given moment and ask them to help you? Can you say to them, can you help me pick this up? Or move this chair? Or carry this box? Or listen to this. … It doesn't sound that difficult, but the courage comes in being willing to show your vulnerability (I need help) to others in a very direct and simple way. … That may be the hardest thing any of us ever have to do. But here's the cool part. Everyone, really everyone, is willing to help, even eager to help you or anyone else. But they just don't know what to do to help. But if they knew, specifically not in general, they all will be glad to do it. And while they are doing it, you get to have some human-to-human interaction. … And this is something you can do right now. No classes to take, no book to read, no sessions to attend. But you gotta have courage to speak up and tell them what you need. Now. … It's win-win. You get some help, they get to help, and everyone feels good." — Jiri Vrba

"I've been learning and practicing Acceptance and Commitment Therapy [ACT] since 2003. I have yet to encounter any experience that cannot be accepted. Although there certainly have been ones that I'm unwilling to accept. But that's my choice. As long as I'm also willing to be responsible for — that is to accept — the consequences of that choice, the peace of mind you mention is available." — Julian McNally

Pain Points are comments on this essay as it appeared originally on Medium.com. They are solely the opinions of the commentators and do not necessarily reflect the views of the book author or publisher.

AFTERWORD

Last Thoughts

Why I created this book

There you go. Thank you for the gift of your time as you've read about my chronic pain journey. It was a big job to get here to the end.

By rights, I should not have been able to create this book. As a chronic pain sufferer, my life is full of challenges. The things most people do easily — like walking — are my bane. I deal with pain daily. As I age, I feel as though I might be falling more and more behind. It's even tough to think when you are in chronic pain, let alone compose a book on it. The pain can overwhelm you, pricking and pounding your psyche. There were times creating this book when I didn't feel well enough to stick with it. I just had to write some days off rather than write.

But, over time, I hung in there. I like to think I'm a good writer and editor, but this book is mostly a result of persistence, perseverance, and perspiration. I hope it gives you insight into the chronic pain experience and inspires you to take on what life has thrown your way with resolve, resilience, and relief.

What kept me going during the hard days? I envisioned other sufferers anxious for answers and feeling alone in their pain. I wanted to help them ease their pain. I hate when people say, "if I can help just one person, then it was worth it." I want to help many more — many, many more. If this book has helped you, I'm gratified. Please leave a review on Amazon and spread the word to family and friends.

My motivation to create this book is summed up by a saying on a freestanding plaque from Amazon my middle daughter gave me for my last birthday. I hope it applies to you:

SOMEBODY OUT THERE NEEDS YOUR WRITING.

Sources of Solace

*Turn to these resources for more information
about living in chronic pain*

You can connect with those who grasp what chronic pain is really like.

With pain support groups, you can find others who understand how devastating chronic pain can be because they're living it or have lived it. It heals to share with others, to feel seen and heard, to be understood.

There are online organizations that offer information, insight, and inspiration about pain. At least two of them facilitate get-togethers among pain sufferers, so people can share what they're going through and swap coping skills, building what "pain warriors" call their "pain toolbox." (See chapter 31.) A third offers resources to learn about chronic pain.

U.S. PAIN FOUNDATION

uspainfoundation.org or painconnection.org
This organization is the leader in bringing attention to and providing services for the chronic pain community.

It gets involved with policy and data gathering about pain, including surveying sufferers.

It publishes magazines within its Invisible Project, including profiles of pain sufferers dealing with a variety of conditions, such as diabetes. It conducts webinars and creates videos to help those in pain.

Its most valuable activity, however, is Zoom support groups offered almost daily through its Pain Connection program.

Via Zoom, pain warriors come together to talk about their conditions and focus on such questions as, "What do you do to deal with flare-ups?"

There are national groups, state groups, and specialized ones, such as an LGBTQ+ gathering and one for veterans.

The groups offer chances for attendees to share their burden of pain and to learn about strategies for dealing with it.

U.S. Pain Foundation is clear that the groups do not provide therapy or medical care. They are led by peer facilitators, whom I've found to be welcoming and warm.

CHRONIC PAIN ANONYMOUS (CPA)

chronicpainanonymous.org

CPA is a 12-step-based organization whose mission is to help chronic pain sufferers.

It does this primarily through meetings via Zoom, online, or face-to-face in groups in various cities.

I've attended a CPA group called Chronically Creative, during which attendees do fun hobbies that distract from pain. As with other support groups, I received a warm welcome as a senior newcomer.

CPA does have a nondenominational religious aspect through its 12-step approach, which is similar to other 12-step groups like Alcoholics Anonymous. The third step of CPA, for example, is, "[We have] made a decision to turn our will and our lives over to the care of God as we understood Him."

Surveys of CPA members show that the program improves a sense of belonging, group support, mental well-being, spiritual well-being, and social connections. (See chapter 26.)

AMERICAN CHRONIC PAIN ASSOCIATION (ACPA)

acpanow.com

The ACPA advocates and offers resources for people in pain. Its activities include:

The ACPA App

Available for iOS and Android, it is a portal to ACPA content and resources that educate people about pain.

ACPA — Stanford Resource Guide to Chronic Pain Management

This is a thorough guide to chronic pain and its treatments published in cooperation with Stanford University's Division of Pain Medicine and Pain Management Center.

Chronicle

ACPA's quarterly e-magazine features articles on various aspects of chronic pain, such as "Finding Strength and Gratitude After a Life-Altering Accident" and "The Power of Self-Care for Pain Relief."

Videos

The ACPA app and website feature videos about pain, including the three-part Family Matters series, which "discusses the issues loved ones face and offers suggestions for keeping the whole family happier and more functional when chronic pain is an unwelcome guest in the home."

The most important message of all these groups is to seek support if you or a loved one is in chronic pain.

Share your story with others in similar circumstances.

Educate yourself through publications and videos.

Seek the solace you need.

OTHER ONLINE RESOURCES FOR PAIN SUFFERERS

- International Association on the Study of Pain (IASP) (iasp-pain.org)

- American Academy of Pain Medicine (AAPM) (painmed.org/american-pain-society/)

- National Pain Advocacy Center (NPAC) (nationalpain.org)

- Facebook and Reddit have active chronic pain support groups. I'm told X does also.

RESOURCES FOR COMMON PAIN CONDITIONS

Arthritis and joint pain

- Arthritis Foundation (arthritis.org)

- Harvard Health Publishing
  (health.harvard.edu/pain/chronic-inflammation-and-your-joints)

- MedlinePlus (medlineplus.gov/jointdisorders.html)

- Mayo Clinic
  (mayoclinic.org/diseases-conditions/osteoarthritis/symptoms-causes/
  syc-20351925)

- WebMD (webmd.com/pain-management/joint-pain)

- "What are some common causes of chronic joint pain?"
  (medicalnewstoday.com/articles/chronic-joint-pain)

Back pain

- National Spine Health Foundation (spinehealth.org)

Cancer pain

- National Cancer Institute (cancer.gov)

- CanCare Cancer Support Groups (cancare.org/services/support-groups)

- American Cancer Society (cancer.org and cancercare.org)

- Cancer Support Community (cancersupportcommunity.org)

Fibromyalgia

- National Fibromyalgia Association (fmaware.org)

- American College of Rheumatology
  (rheumatology.org/patients/fibromyalgia)

- National Institute of Arthritis and Musculoskeletal and Skin Diseases
  (niams.nih.gov/health-topics/fibromyalgia)

- Johns Hopkins Medicine
  (hopkinsmedicine.org/health/conditions-and-diseases/fibromyalgia)

- Cleveland Clinic (my.clevelandclinic.org/health/diseases/4832-fibromyalgia)

- Mayo Clinic
  (mayoclinic.org/diseases-conditions/fibromyalgia/symptoms-causes/
  syc-20354780)

Migraine

- American Migraine Foundation (americanmigrainefoundation.org)

- National Headache Foundation (headaches.org)

- Coalition for Headache & Migraine Patients (CHAMP) (headachemigraine.org)

Myalgic encephalomyelitis/chronic fatigue syndrome (ME/CFS)

- Open Medicine Foundation (OMF) (omf.ngo)

- "ME/CFS Basics" (cdc.gov/me-cfs/about/index.html#cdc_disease_basics_res-resources)

- "Advancing ME/CFS Research" (nih.gov/research-training/medical-research-initiatives/ advancing-mecfs-research)

Neck pain

- Cleveland Clinic (my.clevelandclinic.org/health/symptoms/21179-neck-pain)

- American Association of Neurological Surgeons (aans.org/patients/conditions-treatments/neck-pain/)

Neuropathic pain

- Cleveland Clinic (my.clevelandclinic.org/health/diseases/15833-neuropathic-pain)

- American Academy of Neurology (youtube.com/watch?v=JSBkQtuokJQ)

Please note: Inclusion in Sources of Solace does not constitute endorsement by the author or publisher of any advice, organization, website, product, or service. The list is not meant to be complete; use your internet search skills to seek out more resources. Beware of quacks and scams. Always check with a qualified physician before starting or ending any healthcare regime.

Thank You

My deep thanks to the talented people who contributed to *Chronic Pain Chronicles: Insightful and inspiring stories of resolve, resilience, and relief.*

–Randall H. Duckett, author, editor, and chronic pain sufferer

Associate Editor: **Becky Menn-Hamblin**

Designer: **Katherine Schweiger**

Cover Designer: **Barry Armstrong**

Consulting Editor (and editor of Medium's *Wise & Well* e-publication, in which versions of several of the chapters in *Chronic Pain Chronicles* first appeared): **Robert Roy Britt**

And my appreciation to the scores of people living in chronic pain, experts, study authors, and other sources who are profiled or quoted.

Their insights will help the 60 million other American adult sufferers to learn more about chronic pain, help them feel less alone, and inspire them to take charge of their conditions.

Chronic Pain Chronicles is available as a printed book or ebook from Amazon. Please consider gifting it to pain sufferers among your family and friends.

Thank you for reading *Chronic Pain Chronicles.*

About the Author

Randall H. Duckett is a journalist and lifelong chronic pain sufferer.

He has an inherited disease that caused his bones and joints to deform, leading to osteoarthritis throughout his body. He has had eight joint replacements (both hips twice, both knees, and both shoulders) as well as had his ankles fused. He wrote *Chronic Pain Chronicles: Insightful and inspiring stories of resolve, resilience, and relief* to help the hundreds of millions of people worldwide who, like him, suffer from enduring hurt.

Duckett's journalism and marketing career spanned three decades during which he created, wrote for, and edited scores of magazines and other media for such audiences as high school and college students, healthcare providers and consumers, and travelers. He has authored articles for national publications like *National Geographic Traveler*, *USA Today*, and *AARP: The Magazine*.

After being forced into retirement by disability, he turned his vocation into a pastime to distract himself from his pain. In the early 2020s, he wrote, edited, and published a book on writing called *Seven Cs: The Elements of Effective Writing* (available on Amazon as an ebook or soft-cover book). Following that, he has written dozens of essays on pain and other subjects for Medium.com. He is also the co-author (with his wife, Maryellen Kennedy Duckett or MeK) and editor of travel guides *100 Secrets of the Smokies* and *100 Secrets of the Carolina Coast*.

Randall H. Duckett lives with his wife and family in the Philadelphia area.

www.ingramcontent.com/pod-product-compliance
Lightning Source LLC
Chambersburg PA
CBHW070759280326
41934CB00012B/2982